Mindfulness
for Migraines

An Emergency Physician's Perspective on
Headache Management and Prevention

Ben C Chill, MD

Print ISBN: 978-1-66783-546-4
eBook ISBN: 978-1-66783-547-1

TABLE OF CONTENTS

PART I: IDENTIFYING THE PROBLEM

PART II: IDENTIFYING THE TRIGGERS

PART III: IDENTIFYING THE SOLUTIONS

INTRODUCTION

I was nine years old when I experienced my first migraine. The combination of pain and fear has made that memory a dark fixture in the back of my mind. It was evening, and all of my siblings were home, making a ruckus. Though the chaos was probably typical of that time in my life, it seemed to be a bit louder and more aggressive than usual. I remember starting to feel a dull ache behind my eyes. My mother gave me something chewable, probably Tylenol, and told me to lay down. The pain kept getting worse, throbbing rhythmically, and the light was hurting my eyes. I started to cry. My mother patiently took a rag, soaked in cold water, and pressed it to my forehead. She lay down with me on our shabby, brown couch in the living room and rubbed my neck and back until I fell asleep. My mother wasn't a doctor or a nurse, nor did she have any medical training. She was a parent and a teacher. A sufferer of migraines herself, she understood that medicine alone is not always enough.

Many years and countless headaches later, I am still working on internalizing that lesson. I am an emergency medicine physician with experience in several different hospital systems, multiple emergency departments, as well as urgent care and telehealth. Prior to returning for my post-baccalaureate education, I worked in the mental health field for over 10 years with children and adults diagnosed with developmental disabilities and mental illness. My work in the social services arena combined with formal medical training have led me down the path of utilizing multiple techniques to manage my own headaches.

As an ER doctor, it is my job to identify and address all types of potentially dangerous conditions. We are trained to manage an incredibly broad spectrum of pathology, as pretty much anything can come through our doors at any time. Headaches are one of the top five most common complaints in the emergency department with about four million patients a year in the United States coming into the ER for a headache – and many millions more in outpatient settings.

Of course we must first eliminate dangerous conditions such as stroke or meningitis but in the vast majority of cases, the patient is indeed simply suffering from a bad headache and attempts to treat it at home have failed. If you have ever felt pain on this level, I can definitely relate. You may have even gone to doctors and specialists and tried countless therapies and yet still suffer terribly. I have personally gone down this bumpy road myself and despite my experience and medical education, I found that I was still succumbing to increasingly debilitating headaches. This is why I am always looking for better ways to manage pain.

There are multiple nonmedicinal treatment options available for migraines including mindfulness, biofeedback and cognitive behavioral therapy (CBT). Biofeedback is performed by specialists using techniques such as electroencephalography (EEG) or heart rate monitoring. The goal is to provide immediate feedback to patients about their symptoms using their physiologic responses, thus allowing some control over otherwise unconscious behaviors through education and awareness. Research shows that there are small, but significant improvements in headache symptoms, duration, and frequency with this treatment and it can also help to ease underlying anxiety and depression (Nestoriuc et al, 2008).

Cognitive behavioral therapy is a psychological intervention that utilizes problem-based strategies to address issues involving emotions, thoughts, and beliefs. It combines multiple elements of therapy, and uses a systemic approach to address patient concerns. With headaches, therapists will typically seek out any underlying thoughts or issues related to migraine triggers, such as anxiety or sleep deprivation. A number of studies have been conducted evaluating the effects of CBT for migraines with a moderate level of evidence supporting its use (Pérez-Muñoz et al 2019). Non-pharmacologic management techniques including CBT and mindfulness have been shown to reduce headache intensity as well as lead to improvements in some underlying triggers (Probyn et al, 2017). There are definitely some great potential benefits to a comprehensive approach including a decrease in medication reliance, and a more fundamental understanding of the disease. Many of these interventions can be performed in conjunction with medication management, patient education, and mindfulness.

For many years now, I have been practicing mindfulness-based meditation for a variety of reasons. It has been shown to increase relaxation, productivity, and happiness, as well as countless other health benefits (Van Dam et al, 2018); it has even been proven to be useful in managing pain. While this modality has not been extensively studied specifically for this purpose, there has been a growing body of evidence showing the positive effects of meditation on migraines (Gu et al, 2018, Seminowicz et al, 2020, Wells et al, 2020). Many people suffer from intermittent or chronic pain, and while none of these modalities will make your pain suddenly dissipate the first time you meditate, my goal with this book is to provide you with some tools that may address the underlying contributors to these symptoms. Stress, anxiety, and sleep deprivation are some of the most common culprits known to trigger and exacerbate pain.

This book is divided into three general sections. In the first segment, I will aim to explore the underlying problem. What is a headache? Why do we experience pain in the way that we do? Perhaps most importantly, I will make some recommendations on when it might be a good idea to seek emergency treatment. The second part of the book focuses on the underlying triggers that are often associated with headaches. Some of these include anxiety, stress, sleep deprivation, and dietary issues. Finally, I will discuss some of the ways we can manage our headaches, in particular by focusing on trigger identification, education, and prevention.

Throughout the book are a series of mindfulness modules aimed at addressing pain, triggers, or areas of self-help. If you have never practiced mindfulness in the past, please do not worry or feel intimidated in the least. These are designed to be short, very basic, and easy to follow guided meditation sessions that will hopefully assist you with a number of the goals we will identify throughout this book. I recommend reading them in the order they are laid out first, as they relate to a particular chapter or subject, but feel free to review them more than once, or in any order that works for you. You may get the impression that there is some repetitiveness to these modules. That is no mistake. It is the very act of repetitive practice that allows these techniques to be successful, and for you to properly utilize them in your daily life. By actively participating, practicing, and applying the included modules and the recommended lifestyle changes, you will become better equipped to address and reduce the number and severity of your headaches. True progress takes time and effort. Please keep in mind that making small, sustainable changes is the best way to achieve lasting success.

Mindfulness Module 1: Introduction to Mindfulness

Mindfulness is all about being in the present. It is very natural that we spend much of our time ruminating about the past, thinking about all of the things that we wish we could have done differently, or worrying about what the future might bring, and what steps we need to take to prevent potential issues from arising. The inevitable result is that our present is often filled with stress, pain, or anxiety; we are overwhelmed by both the concerns for the past and the future. How many times have you found yourself lying in bed awake at night with this exact problem? The goal of this process is to find a way to focus your attention on the here and now without getting bogged down in all of our day-to-day concerns. By being present, you will find that there are valuable tools which can be applied to all sorts of areas of your life, including headaches. Try to follow along with the directions of these modules, but please do not judge yourself harshly if you feel like you're not doing it correctly. There is no such thing. The very act of being here and trying to create a better mindset for yourself is an amazing start.

If this is your first time meditating, you will notice that it is very easy for your mind to wander off during these modules. That is perfectly natural. When you notice this has happened, please just acknowledge the thought in a nonjudgmental way. It is absolutely normal for your brain to move from thought to thought. So when you observe this happening, simply redirect yourself by gently bringing your mind back to the present task. For the time you are doing these modules, try to keep the mindset that this is your only responsibility in this moment. For just a few minutes, give yourself permission to place everything else on hold. You will be better suited for all of your other obligations like your work or family, if you can first bring yourself to a healthy and centered place. The first few times you attempt this will likely be very challenging. In fact, even the thousandth time you do this, you may occasionally find yourself feeling almost the same way. However, the more you try, the easier it will become to redirect yourself to where you want to be.

Meditation can be done under any circumstances and in any location. However, for optimal success, I would recommend finding a quiet place where you can sit down in a comfortable and upright position. Of course, this is not always possible, and that is ok. I have often sat in my car in the hospital parking lot to do a pre-shift meditation. Sitting in a waiting room, or on the train or bus waiting for your stop, are all acceptable alternatives. Once again, there is no wrong way to do this. The key is simply to make use of whatever circumstances you have rather than finding an excuse not to try. So wherever you may find yourself at this time, get settled in a comfortable position. Take a nice, slow, deep breath. Soften the muscles of your face, your forehead, the area between your eyes, and unclench your jaw. Keep your spine straight, but with loosened muscles in your neck and back.

Now, at your own pace, notice the breaths entering and exiting through your mouth and nose. Observe the rise and fall of your chest with each breath. Notice how inhaling expands both your chest and abdomen, *and exhaling settles them back down. You will now begin to identify these breaths by the words, "In" and "Out."*

"In," take a breath in, and "Out," let it out.

"In," take a breath in, and "Out," let it out.

Pause here to continue practicing this "In and Out" breathing for at least one full minute if possible – longer if you like. Feel free to close your eyes to increase your focus during this time.

Now you can start to relax your attention on your breathing and return to your natural rhythm. How did it feel to focus on your breathing? Don't worry if your thoughts fluttered around or if you had difficulty attending to the task the whole time. The important thing is that you are making an effort to be present. It may not seem like much, but that is the very essence of meditation. I hope that this determination will plant the seed for a budding success. You are now one step closer to your goals.

PART I: IDENTIFYING THE PROBLEM

CHAPTER 1:
What is a Headache?

Headaches are a complex group of symptoms which form a neurologic disorder that affects millions of people worldwide. Even in this day and age, we don't fully understand how they happen or why some people seem so much more prone to headaches than others. Genetics, nerve and blood vessel abnormalities, and even gender all likely play a role. Women seem to be affected disproportionately, with more than double the incidence of headache syndromes than men, though people of every race, ethnicity, age, and gender suffer from headaches (Vetvik et al, 2017).

For a long time, we thought that perhaps blood vessel malformations in the brain were the main factor. This was called the vasogenic theory, and was favored in the medical community until as recently as the 1980s. The general thinking at the time was that inadequate blood flow was the primary cause of headache development, and could explain certain odd symptoms such as aura in migraines, which I will discuss later on. These blood vessels often run side-by-side with associated nerves, which leads to the neurovascular theory of headaches. This theory suggests that it is the interaction of both blood vessels and sensitive nerve endings that can cause a vicious cycle of pain (Kojic et al, 2013).

There are several nerve structures in the brain that have been of great interest to clinicians as targets for treatment (Robbins et al, 2016). For many years, specialists have used anesthetic agents directed towards these nerves with moderate success. Many other parts of the autonomic nervous system have been thought to play a role as well. This is the body's main control system involved in moderating a large number of functions, including heart rate, digestion, and sexual arousal. Multiple nerve pathways are engaged in this process, and it is heavily activated in the fight or flight response as well as our capacity to feel pain.

Genetics certainly play a role as well, and it is very common to be able to trace at least a little bit of family history of headache disorders. In my own family, my mother and uncle, as well as several of my siblings, all suffer from migraines. In a few rare cases, scientists have been able to pinpoint specific genes that are associated with the disorder. However, most common versions of headaches are thought to have multiple genes involved, and several dozen have already been isolated (Sutherland et al, 2019).

Of the most common headache types are tension headaches and migraines, though there are many other forms as well, such as cluster headaches and sinus pain. Tension headaches are typically felt on both sides of the head, with pressure-like sensations, often described as feeling like a band stretched across the forehead. These can be uncomfortable, to be sure, but are not particularly dangerous. Tension headaches are also usually not quite as debilitating as some of the other headache variants, including migraines. Sinus headaches are somewhat obvious based on their name, and involve pain that can result from sinus congestion or infection. This can be triggered by colds, allergies, or anything that can cause localized inflammation. Pain is generally felt along the sinuses, which are located behind the forehead and upper face. Often, treating the underlying cause is the best way to resolve these issues.

Cluster headaches are a bit of an odd entity. These overlap with migraines to a certain degree in that they are usually felt on only one side of the head, and the symptoms are often severe and recurrent. The peculiar part of cluster headaches is that they can be associated with congestion, tearing of the eye, or even swelling on one side of the face. They can last anywhere from 15 minutes to three hours. Their namesake comes from their tendency to occur in clusters of short attacks, even multiple times on the same day. There appears to be more than double the amount of men affected as women, which stands in stark contrast to most other headache disorders. The current science implicates the nervous system and the trigeminal nerve in particular as possible causes of this disorder. Both cluster headaches and migraines have been shown to share some of the same biochemical pathways which could explain the similarities in pain and treatment. Even with all of the data, we are still unsure about the exact mechanism of cluster headaches. Many of the standard therapies are effective, but we know that providing high-flow oxygen is often successful in treating these attacks. However, despite some commonalities in the diseases, this technique does not seem to help with migraines (Guo et al, 2019).

While there is a wide range of individual experience, migraines come in two major varieties: migraines with aura and migraines without aura. The more common of the two are migraines without an aura, and these are typically described as a throbbing pain felt on one side of the head. The pain pulsates, and can often involve photophobia, or light sensitivity, and may be associated with nausea and vomiting. Mood changes, difficulty concentrating, and congestion are very common complaints for these types of migraines. When I first read about these, many years after my first headache, I felt like I could have fallen right out of the textbook. It also made me feel oddly reassured that so many people were going through exactly the same thing that I had been feeling for so long.

Migraines with an aura may have similar symptoms, but the differentiating characteristic is that they can also be preceded by other sensory or muscle involvement called auras. These auras most commonly manifest as visual disturbances like flashers or floaters. However, less commonly, other odd symptoms can occur, such as paresthesia, (pins and needles), muscle weakness, or even inability to speak (Goadsby, 2012). In fact, people who have migraines with an aura can often experience just the aura itself, without any accompanying pain! The mechanism likely involves genetic predisposition and numerous possible triggers.

Both types of migraines may be preceded by a prodrome phase. This is a period of a day or two prior to the onset of headache when you may experience some nonspecific symptoms such as nausea, constipation, diarrhea, or irritability. Only about 50% of migraine sufferers experience these, and they are not always associated with a migraine, making it difficult to rely on as a specific predictor of headache onset. Some people also experience a postdrome phase. This is a period of a day or two after the actual headache, where you may feel tired and worn out, with diminished energy or even depression-like symptoms. While I do not typically experience visual or sensory auras, I am very well acquainted with both the prodromal and postdromal phases.

Regardless of the type of headache you have, or even the specific symptoms you experience, there is a large overlap in the actual triggers that cause them. From a medical perspective, treating the root source is always the better option. For example, I may note that a patient in the emergency department has very high blood pressure and a rapid heartrate. With no further information, one might think that these abnormal vital signs must be the reason the patient came to the ER in the first place. But if I were to tell you that this patient is 18 years old and she just broke her leg while skateboarding, suddenly you would see this person in an entirely different light. I would obviously not give her blood pressure medication. While her blood pressure and heart rate may improve as a result, this would do absolutely nothing to address the reason they are elevated in the first place; her severe discomfort. Instead, I would treat the underlying cause, the pain of her broken leg, and step back and watch her blood pressure and heart rate return to normal.

This is exactly what I mean when I say sometimes it's better to treat the underlying issues. If the pain you are experiencing is caused by sinus congestion, providing supportive care and, in some circumstances, antibiotics might be the best method of addressing this type of headache. However, as migraines and other types of headaches have such a convoluted and multifactorial pathophysiology, it is not always as simple as treating the underlying cause. And so, we are left with broad pain management techniques, and a number of different types of headache-specific medications, which may work better or worse depending on the person, situation, and history. In addition, we can use our minds, bodies, and actions to address the common triggers involved in all of these processes, including stress, anxiety and sleep disorders. Sometimes, it is just about having the right perspective that can give you the strength you need to overcome your pain.

Mindfulness Module 2: Headache Relief

In this module, we will go over some basic techniques you might find helpful when suffering from a headache. Sometimes you just need a little relief. Though we will review headache triggers like anxiety in greater detail later on, keep in mind that a headache can elicit its own anxiety, which can then lead to an exacerbation of the pain. So give yourself permission to find some relaxation and peace as we move forward. If you are not actively in pain right now, that could actually serve to benefit you. By practicing these techniques when you are able to devote your full attention, you can capitalize on these benefits later on when you really need them.

Take a moment to find a comfortable position. You may lie down or stay seated if that feels right for you. Really settle into the space beneath you. Now relax your eyes. Take a slow, deep breath. We will start by focusing your attention on your head, beginning with the scalp, and then move along in a downward progression. Take your time, read slowly, and try to pause at each location to really concentrate on any sensations that you may be aware of.

Notice the way the top of your hair, or scalp feels against the air around you. Does it feel warm? Perhaps it feels cool? Do you notice any tingling? Is there any air movement you can detect? If you feel nothing, that's ok. Just think, "No sensation" and continue.

Now, move your attention to your ears. How do they feel right now? Do you notice any temperature sensation here? Can you feel any tingling? Perhaps an itch or maybe a dull ache? If you feel nothing, just think again, "No sensation."

Focusing now on your forehead, try to relax any muscles you may be straining; let your eyebrows rest comfortably. Do you notice any warmth or coolness there? Any tingling or pain? If you feel nothing, again, just think, "No sensation."

Shift your attention to your eyes and temples. Release the tension in the muscles between your eyes, and if you are squinting, let your eyes relax. Use your fingers to gently caress the areas over your eyes and temples as a physical reminder that it is ok to let go of that tension. Do you feel any heat or coolness over these areas? Any pain or other sensations?

Now focus on your nose and mouth. Allow the muscles in this area of your face to completely relax. Unclench your jaw. Notice if there are any temperature changes or tingling here. Any sensation of pain? If nothing, please think, "No sensation," and move down.

Begin to focus on your neck now. Allow yourself to soften these muscles, and rotate a little forward, with your chin towards your chest. Then move your left ear over in the direction of your left shoulder. Now, bring your head back towards the center while your head leans toward your back with your face to the sky. And complete the rotation by bringing your right ear to your right shoulder, then back to the center.

Great, now do this again, but in the opposite direction. Start with your chin to your chest before moving your right ear to your right shoulder. Now bring your head back to center while facing the sky, and bring your left ear to your left shoulder. Then return to the center in a resting, comfortable position with your neck straight, but relaxed.

Finally, pay some attention to your shoulders. Relax the muscles there, and rotate them a little bit, letting go of any tension that you may have been holding onto. Do you notice any warmth or coolness in your neck or shoulders? Any other sensations? If there is nothing, that is ok, just think, "No sensation."

Now you may begin to relax your attention on your feelings in your head, neck, and shoulders at this time. I hope that you have begun to feel a little bit better and more relaxed. Sometimes, even such a simple idea as identifying the feelings and sensations we are experiencing, can provide a break in the cycle of pain we are going through. Scanning the muscles involved one group at a time can allow those tensions to recede. Feel free to come back to this module to practice some of these techniques whenever you need a little relief.

Chapter 2:

When to go to the Emergency Department

B efore going any further, it is crucial that I take a moment to remind the reader that while I may be a board-certified doctor, I am in no way able to diagnose you through this medium, and would strongly urge you to seek rapid medical attention for your symptoms if you are uncertain as to their cause. If this is the first time you have ever had a headache, or if it is significantly different than your typical pain, this can certainly be an indication for a more thorough investigation. Although most headaches are not dangerous, my training in emergency medicine has taught me to look out for red flags, which can be a sign of a more sinister pathology. I will go through a few of the major warning signs that we look for in the emergency department, but by no means is this a comprehensive list.

Fever, when accompanied by a headache, is one of the most concerning symptoms. A fever implies the likelihood that there is an associated infection. When these two symptoms are present in isolation, it can be a sign of meningitis. This is especially worrisome when accompanied by neck stiffness, vomiting, and sensitivity to light. That being said, meningitis is a relatively rare infectious cause of headache symptoms, and if there is another obvious source, such as an ear infection or strep throat, which are much more common infectious causes of headache. If the fever is accompanied by cough, congestion, and muscle aches, then it is considerably more likely to be a flu-like syndrome than a rare dangerous pathology. However, if you are unsure, or you are experiencing one of the less common, but frightening signs of meningitis including new seizure activity, confusion, or a neurologic problem like muscle weakness on one side, then this is certainly one of those times to get an emergency evaluation.

The next factor I want to address is timing. The pace at which a headache develops and progresses may be another red flag to look out for. When a patient in the emergency department can tell me the exact time their headache began, it always gives me pause. This generally means there was a sudden onset of symptoms, which can be a sign of danger. More typically of non-lethal causes of headaches are a slow and gradual worsening of symptoms. A headache that is sudden in onset, especially if the initial pain was at its peak at the moment it began, can be a sign of a subarachnoid hemorrhage (SAH). This is a type of bleeding that occurs between layers of the tissue covering the brain. It can occur as a result of a physical injury, or spontaneously from a ruptured aneurysm. Any sort of traumatic event can cause bleeding, and if you have a headache associated with trauma or passing out, even briefly, get an immediate assessment.

I remember one particularly busy day in the emergency department when we had two patients with subarachnoid bleeding at the same time. One was an elderly woman who had fallen out of bed. She was taking a blood thinner, which placed her at higher risk for these types of injuries. The other was a very well-built man in his early 40s. He had been working out at the gym, pushing himself to increase the weights, when he developed a sudden, terrible headache while lifting. He had no other risk factors for bleeding. For months afterward, I found myself paranoid and overly cautious in the gym! The key here is that anyone can potentially be at risk.

Symptoms of subarachnoid hemorrhage can sometimes be tricky to separate out from those of other types of head injuries like a concussion. Typically, SAH symptoms will be more sudden in onset, so if you note that you are having mild symptoms a few days later, you are more likely to be dealing with a concussion or post-concussion syndrome. This is often accompanied by blurry vision, nausea, headaches, and the disturbing sensation of feeling not quite yourself. To be sure, it is not always the easiest diagnosis to make, so if you have a traumatic injury and don't feel well, this warrants at least a thorough physical exam by a trained professional.

It is important to be on the lookout for any factor that could place you at higher risk of bleeding. Some people have genetic predispositions to clotting disorders. Often, there is a strong family history of such things. While some of these disorders create a higher danger of developing blood clots, others, such as hemophilia or low platelets, increase the likelihood of bleeding as well. There are also some medications that may place you at greater risk for bleeding such as "blood thinners." Low-dose aspirin may marginally raise this possibility, but is not considered to be particularly dangerous. However, any of the more potent blood thinning agents which are given to treat blood clots, irregular heartbeats, or mechanical heart valves could place you at a greater risk. If you have a headache, especially an atypical one for you, and you are taking a blood thinner, please seek medical attention immediately.

Though stroke is exceedingly rare in younger individuals, there are some occasions in which it does occur. It can happen after minor trauma, or even spontaneously due to blood clots or bleeding. Patients may present with or without neurologic changes like facial droop or weakness on only one side, or may only have headache or neck pain. The risk is higher with anything that can increase clotting risk in general, such as recent surgery, trauma, pregnancy, or family history. Because of how rare these episodes are, and the vagueness with which they can present, they are also very challenging to diagnose.

This can all sound quite frightening, but before you start running to your local emergency department based on your migraine symptoms, I would like to offer a little reassurance. If you have a headache that is very similar to ones you have experienced in the past, with a comparable rate of onset and intensity, then it is very unlikely to be life-threatening. Your personal headache experience matters more than any description you read in a book or on a website, and is one of the first things I ask about in the emergency department. For example, if you suffer regularly from migraines, and often have visual disturbances such as flashers or floaters, then experiencing these types of symptoms is not likely to be dangerous. However, if you have dealt with headaches many times in the past, and now you are having a visual disturbance for the very first time, you need an evaluation.

There are also some headaches that may not always need an emergency department visit, but should certainly receive urgent evaluation. If you have relatively new and progressive headaches, especially in the morning when you first wake up, this can be a sign of cancer. If these headaches are accompanied by weight loss, night sweats, fatigue, or you never had a headache before and now you have symptoms going on for weeks or months, I urge you to discuss this with your physician. If you already have a diagnosis of cancer or are known to have a weakened immune system, this could have similar ramifications associated with the spread of disease.

Headaches that are new or atypical, particularly in those over the age of 50, should be a cause for concern. Children, especially under the age of 5, do not normally complain of headaches. Unless they have some other illness like a virus, be sure to discuss their headache complaints with their physician. Please take any new deviations from your typical symptoms very seriously and reach out for appropriate medical care. Though this is not an all-inclusive list of the dangerous pathologies that headaches may present, it encompasses some of the more common elements we look for in the emergency department. In summary, remember, if this is a new type of headache for you, or is accompanied by one of the dangerous signs we talked about above, please seek medical assessment as soon as possible.

Module 3: Breathing with a Point

Headaches can be challenging. Finding a way to improve your pain in any way can be a huge blessing. Sometimes, it is not feasible to take medication, or you may have taken the meds, but need some time for them to start working. The goal of this module is to be able to find some relief through purposeful redirection. Though there are many ways to redirect your attention, what is nice about breathing is that no matter where you are, you always have it with you. Therefore, it is a quick and reliable method of focus control. There is also a beauty in the shared commonality that breathing provides. No matter the color of your skin, your age, nationality, or even species. Each and every one of us relies on breathing to provide our bodies with the oxygen we need to survive.

Begin by taking a moment to find a comfortable position. Relax your eyes and really sink into the space around you. You may find that the best position for you is sitting up, leaning back, or even lying down, though be careful to notice if you are getting too sleepy. The most important thing is to situate your body in a way that allows you to relax and clear your mind.

Take a nice, slow, deep breath filling your lungs and expanding your chest. Now slowly exhale and feel whatever tension you may be holding onto start to gradually soften as well. Take another deep breath and hold it for a moment. Now exhale again, slowly, feeling the tension inside you further loosen and release. Now, one more time, take a deep breath in, getting ready to release all the stress and tension inside, and finally, expel that pressure with your breath, slowly, until it is gone.

If you can, bring the pointers of both hands along with your middle fingers to your temples. Gently touch your temples just behind your eyes on both sides and slowly massage first clockwise and then counter-clockwise along with your breaths. With every breath in you will rotate your fingers up and forward, and with every breath out, rotate them down and back. Leave your thumbs resting gently at the angle of your jaw, just below your ears. You are going to time your breaths along with your fingers. If at any point you are feeling out of breath or lightheaded, please relax and return to breathing at your own natural rhythm. So, as you breathe in, rotate your fingers forward and up, and then as you breathe out, switch directions, down and back.

Breathe in, move your fingers forward and up. Breathe out, move your fingers backward and down. Breathe in, forward and up. Breathe out, backward and down. In, forward and up. Out, backward and down. In, forward. Out, backward.

Don't worry if you're not sure if you're moving in the right direction, just alternate along with your breaths.

Breathe in, forward and up. Breathe out, backward and down. In, forward. Out, backward.

You might notice that your mind wanders back to the stressful thoughts of your day, to your pain, or somewhere else completely, but again, don't worry, just acknowledge that your mind is doing what it does best, "thinking," and then gently move back to focus on your breathing and the sensation of your fingers on your skin.

Breathe in, forward and up. Breathe out, backward and down. Breathe in, forward and up. Out, backward and down. In, forward. Out, backward.

Now, you may begin to relax your focus on your breaths, returning to your natural breathing pattern. You may keep your fingers at your temple if that feels right, or you may drop them to your sides or lap in any position that feels good for you. Stay like this for just a moment longer. Take a nice, deep breath in, and for the final time, see if you can breathe out any of the last remaining bits of tension.

Take a moment to consider how you feel. Are you a bit more relaxed then when you began? Does your head hurt a little less? Perhaps there is a small reduction in tension in your neck and jaw. Remember, doing this once is great. It can certainly help to provide some relief. But doing this regularly and aiming to internalize it through regular practice is the best way to maximize your success.

Chapter 3:

Pain

P ain is a much more complicated subject than it first appears. From a medical perspective, we can draw lines and point a finger at the nerves and muscles involved in the sensation of pain, and lots of times, we can see exactly what is causing it. For example, recall the young skateboarder who broke her leg in Chapter 1. The source of her pain is obvious. Your body's sympathetic nervous system possesses a complex network of nerves that communicate at incredibly rapid rates to let your brain know that something is wrong.

As the ground approaches the skateboarder, at an unfortunate angle for her left leg in particular, her nerves are already on the alert. They first try to prevent the injury from occurring at all by having her body move into whatever defensive position it can. In this situation, sadly, it was not fast enough. Immediately upon contact, these nerves inform her brain about what is happening, so that she may begin to respond. Which direction is she falling in, how can she stop herself? What is the best way to minimize the immediate danger? Now that she has fallen, is she still in danger? Or can she take the time to address her injury? In shock, she may not even feel pain right away until her brain acknowledges that it is safe to do so. Evolutionarily speaking, if we did not develop this mechanism of feeling pain, we would not know to protect ourselves in order to prevent or treat injuries.

When I was in my early 20s, I had the misfortune of getting into a motorcycle accident. A truck shifted into my lane, and I instinctively moved over towards the side of the road which was covered in gravel. As I rounded the next bend, I noted that the oncoming traffic light was turning red. I was a novice rider at the time and I tried to brake too hard on the gravel-covered pavement. This caused my motorcycle to slide out from underneath me and began skidding towards the intersection. Everything around me seemed to slow down; sound itself disappeared. I didn't know that I had hurt myself until I finally stopped bouncing on the street and was grateful to find that I was able to stand up. Time and sound returned to normal, and only then did I realize that my left arm felt like it was burning and I could barely move my shoulder. It was very clear where my pain was coming from.

In many other circumstances, the source of your pain may be more difficult to pin down. Abdominal pain is probably one of the most common examples of this that I see in the emergency department. Unfortunately, the nerves in your stomach are not as precise as the ones closer to the skin, and have a very difficult time telling your brain exactly where the source of the pain is. The inherent challenge is that it can come from so many different sources. Appendicitis, urinary tract infections, or a viral illness like a stomach bug are just a few of the vast number of possibilities that can present in much the same way.

Thus, the ER visit for this type of pain typically involves an extensive evaluation consisting of a combination of reviewing medical history and a thorough physical exam. Many times this is accompanied by bloodwork or even imaging to determine the basis of the symptoms. Despite all of that, even after many hours of testing and utilizing the most modern, state-of-the-art technology, we still often fail to diagnose the cause of a patient's pain. This experience is something I am all too familiar with. I would love to tell every patient that I know exactly why they are having discomfort and just how we are going to resolve it. Sadly, we are often left with only the silver lining that it does not appear to be a dangerous or surgical cause, but ultimately both the patient and I are dissatisfied with the lack of a specific diagnosis.

Headaches are much the same. Many of you reading can attest that you suffer from horrible and often debilitating headaches. However, if you or your doctors have decided to pursue radiographic imaging of the brain, most of you will have found largely unremarkable results. CT scans and MRIs with all of their amazing capacity to visualize minute details in the folds of your brain and surrounding blood vessels still come up short in the majority of headache cases. Once again, you are left with the security that it is unlikely dangerous, but with the inherent dissatisfaction that comes with not having a specific reason for your pain.

Even the triggers and their effects can vary widely. Lack of sleep, caffeine intake, stress, and many other factors can be involved. But sometimes, you can experience an excruciating headache, despite having a perfect night's sleep. You can also be very overtired after a terrible night's sleep, and have no headache at all. We are left with an imperfect science and a likely elaborate and multi-faceted disease process. Thus, we attempt to treat whatever underlying issues we can, in the hopes of preventing or diminishing even a few of these headaches.

One of the most common migraine triggers is tension. Life can be extraordinarily stressful. No matter what age you are, or at what stage in life, the body's stress system, activated by cortisol, responds in much the same way. Stress triggers your brain, which releases hormones that stimulate your adrenal glands to produce more cortisol and adrenaline. This can lead to a lot of potentially negative outcomes in your body with elevated levels of stress and inflammation. Working in the field of emergency medicine has forced me to find ways to cope with a high level of stress on a regular basis. Perhaps you work in a tough environment with a challenging supervisor or irritating co-workers. Maybe you are in school and laboring intensively to perform well on exams or term papers. Or perhaps you are retired, struggling financially, or have difficult neighbors. Regardless of your relationship status, income level or stage in life, these stressors may trigger your headaches.

A little bit of stress can actually be a good thing. The Yerkes-Dodson law, published in 1908, presents this as a bell curve. On the far end of the curve, too much stress is noted to lead to a decrease in productivity. This is somewhat intuitive. Think of a student preparing for an extremely important exam. The student's entire career and way of life depend on this one number. She might stay up late studying, drinking coffee after coffee, pushing herself to the limit. But because of the immense pressure, she can barely focus. Her eyes are bloodshot, and she can barely think. Despite all of her efforts, she remains at high risk of failure if she succumbs to the crushing weight of the task. And that is not taking into account the physical and emotional strain that the elevated levels of cortisol may be having on her as well. When she finally takes the exam, the words will be swimming around in her brain, and her cortisol-addled mind will be unable to correctly identify the answers.

Less obviously, on the shallow end of the curve, low levels of stress are associated with a decrease in productivity as well. Why would that be? This may seem counterintuitive on the surface. One might think that if only life were to be completely stress-free, we would be able to achieve so much. While this might work for a short period of time, this is likely far from reality. Imagine an alternate exam, but this time, one that has no impact on the future for this student. If the student knew that the score did not count and would not contribute in any way to her overall grade for the class, this would be an example of too little stress. She may choose to spend her time on something else entirely, and not even bother to prepare, resulting in a miserable failure.

Now consider these circumstances reconfigured one more time with just the right amount of stress. Enough urgency to provide motivation, but not too much to completely incapacitate. Perhaps there is a reasonable quantity of information being tested and adequate time to prepare. This student also has supportive parents and teachers who instill within her the knowledge that while it is important to do well and always try your best, the test represents just one number in the scheme of things. Now our young pupil is in her element. She will work hard and efficiently, without the burden of disproportionate stress, increasing the odds of her ultimate success.

As I noted above, stress can lead to the triggering of the cortisol system, and the physical manifestations of this tension can be the undesired tightening of muscles. From a headache perspective, it is the muscles of the shoulders, neck, face, and jaw in particular that are involved, often with significant overlap. An unfortunate consequence of this is that the resulting headaches can lead to further tension, which leads to a vicious cycle of pain and muscle spasm. So if we can relieve tension, even briefly, it may help to stop the pain cycle providing more long-term relief. Mindfulness can be an amazing resource for this particular problem.

Module 4: Tension Reduction

The goal of this module is to address the tension that results from and causes more muscle spasm, which can lead to worsening headache symptoms. We will first identify the muscles involved, and actively relax them, while also working to maintain an emotional calm. The theory behind the specific location of applied forces in this module is based on the anatomy of some of the nerve structures thought to play a role in migraines. These nerves are sometimes the focus of neurologists and specialists who use anesthetic agents to treat pain. We will apply the same strategy by using your own body and mind to break the pattern causing your headache.

Take a moment to find a comfortable position. Relax your eyes and adjust your body to be as loose and decompressed as possible. Focus on the muscles of your face and neck, and allow them to soften. Beginning with the top of your head and forehead, consciously relax any areas of tension you may feel. If you are furrowing your brow or squinting your eyes, please gently let go of this pressure. Now, moving on to your face, try to relax any tensed muscles, including the area around your mouth and jaw. Unclench your teeth. Bring your attention down to your neck. Feel free to move it gently from side to side and flex up and down before settling on the most comfortable position that works for you.

Now take a nice, slow, deep breath. If you are able, bring your pointer and middle finger from each hand and place them gently on your forehead. You may include your other fingers if that feels right to you. Using as many fingers as you like, softly brush your fingers up and down and side to side along your forehead. Feel for any contracted muscles and remind yourself that it is ok to relax them. Now, move your pointer and middle finger to your temples. Apply light pressure to your skin. With a soft, clockwise motion, begin gently massaging your temples. With every rotation, give yourself permission to release any tension you may have built up over the course of your day.

Now, move your fingers back along your scalp on either side of your head, just above your ears, but this time with a little more pressure. If at any point it is causing you pain or discomfort, please ease up or stop, and imagine the sensation instead. Gliding your fingers even farther back, moving a little bit lower, try to find the bony ridge of your skull an inch or two behind your ears. Let your fingers move further back behind this bone, and settle into a gentle massage of the soft area just behind this ridge.

Moving your hands closer together towards the very back of your head, keep up a soft massaging motion. Feel free to do it as deeply or as lightly as feels right. Continue to move your fingers closer together until they are almost touching.

Finally, using as many fingers as you like, move down to your neck and gently massage up and down. Find any muscles that are still tense and allow yourself to let them go. Continue your movements and take a nice, long, deep breath. Feel free to release your hands to your sides, in your lap, or whatever position feels comfortable for you. If you were just imagining the sensation, relax your focus on your scalp and neck at this time. Take a moment to reflect on how you feel right now. Are you more relaxed? How do the muscles in your neck and face feel? Has the tension ebbed, even just a little? This module, as with any other resource, can provide some tools for headache relief. As is true in all areas of life, different techniques or experiences will have varying degrees of success depending on the individual. Try to take the parts of everything that you learn or encounter that work well for you, and really make them your own.

Part II: Identifying the Triggers

Chapter 4:

Anxiety

Emotions play a very important role in how we perceive pain and how we process information from the world around us. Envision a young man, newly in love and romantically courting the young lady of his dreams. No amount of rain or cold is going to bring down this confident suitor. He is happy as a clam, with a smile plastered all over his beaming face. He can trip and fall, rip his pants, drop all of his belongings into a muddy puddle, or have a high-pressure presentation coming up at work and he will cope with all of these challenges with ease, thanks primarily to his charmed perspective. This is not to say that rose-tinted glasses will protect him from suffering a tragic loss or serious calamity, but it is obvious that being in a better place emotionally can act as a sort of shield of armor, protecting its wearer.

Some days in the emergency department can seem like they drag on forever and there are constant delays with difficult evaluations. Every interaction can seem tedious and more burdensome than the last. Other days can seem remarkably light and flow beautifully, despite having patients and pathologies that are every bit as challenging. The difference between those days may depend on my own mood and perspective. Am I tired? Do I have a headache? Am I hungry? Have I had enough water to drink? Am I just anxious?

Anxiety can be the deciding factor in a potentially stressful scenario. Imagine our young man, no longer in the throes of passionate love, but still getting ready for that high-pressure presentation. His boss and colleagues are all relying on him. If this goes well, not only could this bring the company to the next level, it can mean the very survival of the entire business. If this presentation does not pan out, he may well lose his job, not to mention the respect of his colleagues and boss. Obviously, this is a tremendously demanding situation. Add to that burden the fact that his high-school sweetheart and fiancée has just ended their engagement, and he has been wallowing in self-pity for a week. How can anyone flourish under these miserable circumstances? No doubt the anxiety he feels will be wildly exacerbated in this situation, jeopardizing his ultimate success.

I cannot begin to tell you how often relatively young patients with no medical issues at all come to the emergency department complaining of severe chest pain. They tearfully tell me they are short of breath and have terrifying tingling and numbness to both of their hands and sometimes their feet. Their arms and jaw hurt. The symptoms seem to come up whenever they are studying at night. They are absolutely certain this must be a heart attack at the ripe old age of 22 with no family history or chronic illnesses. It can't possibly have anything to do with the fact that they are in finals season and pushing themselves for days and days cramming for exams and handing in term papers, right? Of course, there are always exceptions, but most of the time, this is a fairly straightforward panic attack.

This is just one of the many classic manners in which anxiety can present itself, and is almost too easy to see when you are looking from the outside in. But fear changes the way you see things too. It has real physical effects that can certainly lead to real physical harm. We already talked about the cortisol stress system and its consequences which are undoubtedly utilized by anxiety as well. Often, these patients will have an elevated heart rate and blood pressure, at least initially, until they calm down. That is a measure of additional strain on their bodies, and certainly could be detrimental if it is ongoing for a prolonged period of time, or even relatively frequently over the course of years. Thus, anxiety can lead to increased tension, depression, sleep deprivation, and generalized inflammation that can all lead to more headaches with worse symptoms. In order to properly address it, we must first recognize that what we are experiencing is actually anxiety.

There are many different types of anxiety that can manifest in ways you might not consider. Social anxiety may occur in any setting involving meeting other people, particularly unfamiliar faces. This can happen at work, school, parties, dates, job interviews, and even shopping for groceries. This has the potential to lead to avoidance of any situation which can lead to discomfort, thereby indirectly limiting success in any of these circumstances. If you are afraid to meet new people, you may find an excuse not to apply for a job that you may be particularly well suited for. This can lead to lost opportunities for income and friendships at work. The negative downstream effects of such a process are easy to imagine.

Though anxiety may come in all shapes and sizes, the central theme is often an irrational fear of some kind of environmental or social interaction. Usually these fears are baseless, but some can appear to be superficially rational, like a fear of heights, snakes, or spiders. These become pathologic when it is obvious to anyone else that you are not in danger, like visiting a zoo and observing a snake behind thick glass. Yet the experience may still cause your heart to race and palms to sweat. Regardless of which form of this disorder you identify with, it can function as a trigger for your headaches. Having a strong social support system and appropriate medical follow up are key to addressing these issues. This can help to augment your ability to not only address the anxiety itself, but may actually assist in preventing and managing the associated headache symptoms that result.

On a personal note, it is not uncommon for me to suffer from anxiety when I am at work. There are some days that can be really tough. Perhaps a colleague has called in sick, and it is particularly busy in the emergency room. The patient volume feels like it is exploding, and some of my patients are actually quite ill. I am juggling orders and trying to be at the bedside of the people who need me the most. As a physician, I need to maintain calm, and direct the management of every patient in my care. It can be quite overwhelming. There are many important methods for maintaining a healthy perspective, but there are three main techniques that I employ to sustain my own serenity during these demanding shifts, and they can be broadly applied to many stressful situations.

1: Self-Triage:

I periodically review each patient under my care, from earliest to newest, skipping to the patients who are sicker and need more immediate attention. This allows me to maintain a grounded perspective, while also staying on top of my game. This doesn't only apply in an emergency department. When you feel like you have too many items on your plate, it is time to take inventory. Trying to focus on everything at once will get you absolutely nowhere.

In today's day and age, the whole world can feel like an emergency department. Life is full of demands on both your time and attention. Whether it is your kids, work, or the million tasks that you have to take care of, there is always something that needs your consideration. Choose the issues that need to be addressed first, and then move on to the next in order of importance. From time to time, review your goals to help you stay on task.

2: Maintain Focus:

Try to focus on only one thing at a time. Many people pride themselves on their ability to multitask. The truth is, we are not particularly good at multitasking. There is a limited amount of working memory available to us at any given time, so we are actually more likely to task switch than to multitask (Skaugset et al 2016). This is not just semantics; it takes an average of 23 minutes to get back to a task once we switch to another (Pattison, 2008). I make every attempt to be as courteous as possible to the nurses, ECG technicians, and other clinical staff members as I politely ask them to wait for a moment as I complete my task. It makes me more efficient and is definitely better for overall patient care.

Whether you are in an office setting or working from home, if you are trying to respond to emails and texts while talking on the phone, your work is going to suffer. Focus on one task to completion and then pick up the next whenever possible. You will notice that your efficiency and effectiveness will improve and you will feel less emotional strain.

3: Take a Break:

When I am feeling overwhelmed, the resulting anxiety can prevent me from making the rapid assessments and quick judgments that are vital to my job. So, perhaps somewhat counterintuitively, this is when I take a break. Not an hour-long lunch break or taking a nap in the on-call room, but just a few minutes to myself. I am fortunate that there is an office right next to the emergency department where I can go to sit down. I take about three minutes at most to pause and breathe. This is a time for myself; a moment to reset. For those brief moments, work does not exist. Once I am done, I find that I am again able to make those difficult, but vital decisions we are called upon to make each day.

The manner in which we handle fear and stressful situations can strongly impact our day-to-day lives, and we know that increased anxiety can be a significant stressor when it comes to pain and migraines (Tang et al, 2005; Peres et al, 2017). Finding better ways to manage these stressors can contribute to an improved understanding of both ourselves and the environment around us. That knowledge is the key to providing us with another mindfulness-based tool to help prevent and treat the underlying issues contributing to headaches.

Module 5: Rapid Reset

I would like to share with you a technique for a quick and vital reset that I perform at work. It can be used anytime, of course, and if you need it while dealing with a difficult child, or a tough interaction with a friend, feel free to apply it however you see fit. The point is really a matter of grounding yourself in the present moment. This allows your worries about the past or concern for the future to melt away for just long enough to re-center yourself.

If possible, find a quiet area, but if this is not an opportune time for that, any space will do. Even if you have to do this walking in a hallway or outside, just do the best you can.

If you are able to, sit down and relax your eyes. Settle into whatever space you chose, and take a deep, slow breath. Now, take a second to look around you. Pick a nearby object to focus on. It can be a coffee mug, your keyboard, a stapler, any object you choose is fine. Notice this object and say to yourself, in your mind, "This is a _____," and insert the name of this object here. So, if you chose a coffee mug, say, "This is a coffee mug."

Great. Then relax your eyes again and take another deep, slow breath.

If you have time, repeat this once or twice, using different objects, but even doing it just once can help you to reset your focus, giving you the ability to be more productive at work, or have more patience if you need it. The logic behind this simple technique stems from the idea that many of the mental and emotional struggles we deal with can pull us in opposing directions. We go back and forth trying to resolve these things, but often, in such a manner as to be less efficient overall. This leaves us feeling unbalanced and strained. By focusing on the mundane, a mug in the example above, allows our minds to become grounded once again. This can give us the strength and fortitude we need to accomplish our goals.

Module 6: Box Breathing

This module is a bit longer and aimed at addressing underlying anxiety that can serve as a trigger to migraines, pain, and general unhappiness. This can cause an unrelenting cycle of self-perpetuation. The stress alone can lead to a hyper-focus on the issue itself, preventing you from finding a solution. The goal here is to find an alternative focus to give your mind and emotions the space and tools they need to recover. The advantage to utilizing breathing for this approach is its accessibility and ready availability.

We are going to use a controlled breathing approach combined with a visualization technique which is geared towards helping you clear your mind and redirect your attention. This will help to activate your body's parasympathetic nervous system, allowing you to naturally relax. If at any point, you begin to feel uncomfortable or short of breath, please return to your natural rate and rhythm of breathing, but continue to follow along by counting your breaths.

Take a moment to find a nice, quiet space and a comfortable position. Settle in to the most relaxed space for your body. Relax your eyes. Take a nice, slow, deep breath in, and slowly let it out. Now, take another, and again, slowly let it out while concentrating on removing any tension you may be holding onto. Now take one more deep breath, releasing it nice and slowly and letting go even further.

Pay attention to the way your breathing makes your chest rise and fall. Breathe in, and your chest rises, and breathe out, it falls. Notice how it makes your abdomen move in and out as well. Now, try to focus *on breathing in through your nose, and out through your mouth. Some people breathe like this naturally, but many of us do not, and it may feel somewhat awkward or a little uncomfortable at first. Take your time and allow your body to gradually adjust.*

Now let your breathing settle down, in through your nose and out through your mouth. Think "In" when breathing in, and think "Out" when breathing out.

1) *Breathe in and think, "In," and breathe out and think, "Out."*

2) *Breathe in and think, "In," and breathe out and think, "Out."*

3) *Breathe in and think, "In," and breathe out and think, "Out."*

Now, increase your control using the following four steps.

1) *You will take a slow breath in through your nose while counting to 4.*

2) *Then you will hold your breath for a count of 4.*

3) *Breathe out through your mouth, counting to 4.*

4) *Hold your breath again counting to 4.*

Imagine you are drawing a box that will contain your anxiety. Breathing in builds the wall up, holding creates the top of the box, breathing out is the wall on the other side, and holding again creates the base of the box.

1) *Breathe in through your nose for a count of 1, 2, 3, 4, and build the first wall of the box.*

2) *Hold your breath for a count of 1, 2, 3, 4, and build the top of the box.*

3) *Breathe out through your mouth for a count of 1, 2, 3, 4, and build the opposite wall.*

4) *Hold your breath again for a count of 1, 2, 3, and 4 creating the base of the box.*

Now repeat this four more times. You can do more if you wish, but try at least four.

Once complete, you may release your attention on the box building and resume breathing in whatever way feels most comfortable for you. Picture the box you've just created. What does it look like? Is it solid or clear? What is it made of? Wood? Metal? Or some other material? Imagine that box, built by the controlled and measured breaths you took, enveloping your anxiety. Watch it as it slowly begins to fade into the background. It is turning into a smoky mist, dwindling away gradually in your mind, along with any remaining anxiety you may have been holding onto, until it is barely visible. Now, it is gone. Take a moment to appreciate the work you did today. Just taking the time to be here and striving for a healthier life is a great step toward handling your anxiety. Even if you don't have time to do a full module, the next time you feel the need, draw one quick box with your breath and see how you feel.

Module 7: Color Breathing

This is another mindfulness module aimed at reducing anxiety using visualization. In this one, we will incorporate our perception of color into our breathing. This will serve to bring an additional layer of focus to our breathing techniques. The overall goal is to direct attention at addressing whatever tension or anxiety you may have built up. These thoughts can weigh you down and hinder your progress, getting in the way of successful relationships, interpersonal communication, and professional success. It is so important to find the time to take for yourself and to learn to let go of these negativities, so that you can move on.

Take a moment to find a quiet space to sit. Close your eyes and settle into the chair or the ground beneath you. Take a deep breath. Soften the muscles of your face, your brow, your mouth, and unclench your jaw. Now breathe naturally, inhaling and exhaling at your own natural pace. Feel the way your chest rises as you breathe in, and settles as you breathe out. Notice the effect that your breathing has on your abdomen. Feel free to place one or both hands on your stomach, and observe how your inhale causes your abdomen to expand as well. Then watch as it settles back as you exhale. It is amazing how many muscle groups are affected by the movements of your breathing.

As you continue to focus, imagine that the air entering your body has a color. Think of a smooth, light blue shade that softly caresses your nostrils as you breathe in, cooling your throat and filling your lungs. When you breathe out, the air is red. A warm, but gentle hue, which emanates from deep within you, pulling all of your tension and anxiety with it.

Breathe in light blue, and breathe out warm red. Breathe in, blue. Then breathe out, red. In, blue. Out, red.

You might notice that your mind has begun to drift; that is ok. Just acknowledge that you are thinking, and gently nudge your thoughts back to the color of your breathing.

Breathe in, light blue, and breathe out, warm red. Breathe in, blue. Then breathe out, red.

Now, imagine this beautiful, blue breath, not only going in through your mouth, and filling your lungs, but entering all of the pores of your body, from the soles of your feet to the top of your head. You breathe that soothing blueness with all of your pores, allowing the healing oxygen to

43

reach every vital part of you. Now when you breathe out from every part of your body, that red, gentle warmth carries with it everything you want and need to let go of.

Breathe in, with your whole being, blue, and breathe out, everywhere, red. Breathe in, with all of your body and soul blue, and let go of everything, red. In, completely blue. Out, everything red.

Now you may begin to let go of your focus on the color of your breathing, and settle back into a natural, normal rhythm. How did it feel to imagine all of your pores breathing? How did it feel to assign a color to the air? This can be a challenging concept, and I encourage you to practice as many times as you need. Letting go of your anxieties and thoughts of emotional or physical pain can really open the doors you might need to allow yourself to heal.

Chapter 5:
Sleep Deprivation

Sleep is one of the most underrated necessities in our lives. On average, people spend approximately a third of their lives asleep, and yet, we understand decidedly little about what sleep is or why we need it. Not to say that there isn't a plethora of research on the topic, but even after millennia of human consideration and decades of formal study, there is still so much to learn. What we do know is that without enough sleep, we make poor decisions, feel less energized, tend to be more moody, and think less clearly (Chunhua et al, 2019). For those of us who are prone to headaches, sleep disturbances can lead to increased frequency of headaches with even more severe and debilitating symptoms (Song et al 2018). I often compare being overtired to being drunk; it's just much less fun. You forget words, slur your speech, lose focus quickly, and are generally unpleasant to be around. You would also be just as dangerous behind the wheel of a car or operating heavy machinery.

David, a friend of mine from college decided that he was going to experiment with purposeful insomnia. Dave had heard that if you stayed up for long enough, you would start to hallucinate. The first

24 hours passed fairly uneventfully. He played guitar, hung out with friends, and seemed like his normal self. However, as Dave closed in on 36 hours, he became increasingly irritable and snappy. After that, he became progressively slower, bleary-eyed, and angry. We all began avoiding direct contact with him as his interpersonal skills and innate charm had almost completely deteriorated by that point. I don't recall exactly how long he made it, though David insisted it was over 48 hours. No, he did not hallucinate. Having witnessed this, I would certainly recommend against conducting this experiment on your own.

Clearly sleep, or lack thereof, plays a huge role in our lives. Without enough of it, we are prone to multiple triggers of headaches and pain, not to mention many other negative impacts on our day-to-day lives. As an emergency medicine doctor, this is a big personal problem for me. I have to work shifts at all hours of the day and night, and it has been one of my greatest challenges to achieve adequate sleep hygiene. So let's take some time to discuss some measures that can help you get a better night's sleep. Ideally, keeping a regular schedule and going to bed at around the same time every night will help your body and mind adjust to getting into the appropriate mental state for sleeping. Once you set this agenda for yourself, you will notice that your body will begin to grow tired and you will have the urge to go to bed at around the same time every day.

Developing good habits is what makes sleep hygiene a success. Create a routine for yourself that works for you. Pick a time that you will stop eating for the day, brush your teeth, change into your night-time attire, and turn off your television. Power down or silence your cell phone as well. I recommend at least an hour off any device, if possible, prior to the time you want to actually be asleep. The lighting from these gadgets as well as the constant influx of attention-grabbing media will doubtlessly inhibit your ability to fall into a restful slumber.

Your body naturally produces a hormone called melatonin. As the environment begins to grow darker, production of melatonin ramps up, making you feel more tired. You can imagine how this would have been very practical from a historic perspective prior to the development of artificial light sources. As the night closes in on morning, the levels of this hormone begin to drop, making you feel less tired. If you are on your phone or watching TV in bed with light directly in your eyes, your melatonin production may be unintentionally inhibited, making it more difficult to fall asleep (Wood et al, 2013).

Your bedroom should be a sanctuary. Thinking of it this way can help you organize it in a way that will be most conducive for sleep. Try not to do any other activities in this room, except for those fitting for bedroom behavior, of course. Removing your television or computer completely and placing them in an alternate location in your home can help maintain this refuge. If you can, ensure that your bedroom is as dark as possible. Just like TV and other devices, outside light can trigger your brain into thinking it is time to be awake.

Keep the room a little on the cool side if that is comfortable for you. You may notice that you feel drowsier in a warm room, and there are several explanations for this. Elevated temperature can cause your blood pressure to lower slightly, which may make you feel tired. It may also cause you to expend more energy to keep cool, causing fatigue. However, it may not be the most ideal way to maintain sleep once you've achieved it. This is likely another circumstance of circadian rhythm playing a role in sleep. As your body shuts down, your internal thermostat decreases as well. As the morning approaches, your body begins to warm up again. This is probably why an overheated room may make it more difficult to remain asleep. Of course, extreme cold will make this difficult as well, so it is really important to carefully control your environment for ideal sleep.

Avoiding alcohol and caffeinated beverages, especially close to bedtime, is also a good idea. These substances activate your mind in ways that are not particularly conducive to restful sleep. Caffeine is an obvious culprit. Whether or not you can fall asleep without apparent difficulty, even after downing an extra-large iced coffee from your favorite cafe, does not mean that your brain isn't all hyped up on caffeine. Even if you fall asleep, that brain activity may impede your sleep from being as restful and restorative as it could have been (Clark et al, 2017). Unsurprisingly, after just one night of poor sleep, you find that you are a bit more tired the next day. So you reach for a little extra coffee to give you a boost. The additional caffeine makes it harder to fall asleep, and before you know it, you're locked into a malicious cycle. Not to mention that the caffeine reliance will also place you at greater susceptibility for caffeine withdrawal headaches (Juliano et al, 2019).

Alcohol is a somewhat less obvious perpetrator. On the surface, you might think that a drink or two will help you sleep, and you may even recall times when you found yourself passing out after a night of drinking. This is completely rational as alcohol is technically a depressant, which means that it acts on receptors in your brain in such a way as to make you sleepier. This leads to some of the related symptoms that we recognize in intoxication, such as slurred speech and delayed reflexes. Despite its inhibitory effects, however, alcohol has been shown to hamper restful sleep, (Ebrahim et al, 2013) and it is associated with many other issues as well, such as liver problems, cancer, dependence, and abuse. There are several stages the body goes through every night when sleeping, including REM sleep. Alcohol can disrupt these patterns, leading to poor sleep and worse outcomes.

Sleep stages are cyclical. Stage 1 of sleep is when your body starts to wind down. Your heartrate slows and your muscles relax. The busy activity of your brain starts to decrease. During stage 2, your body continues to ease and deescalate, your eyes stop moving as much, and your body's internal thermostat decreases. Stage 3 is the slowest stage. Approximately 90 minutes into the cycle is when you start having REM sleep. REM stands for rapid eye movement, and this is the stage when most dreams take place. It is thought that this stage plays an important role in memory consolidation and retention (Klinzing et al, 2019). When you drink, you change the amount of time spent in these cycles, altering it in ways that can diminish restfulness and memory, and can lead to severe sleep disruptions and insomnia (Ebrahim et al, 2013).

Healthy eating habits and regular exercise can also contribute to sleep hygiene (Vitale et al, 2019). The less fatty, sugary, and oily foods you put into your body, the better. Avoid exercising too close to bedtime, because although it may tire you out, it actually causes an increase in the production of endorphins, which stimulate both your body and mind in ways that are amazing, but certainly not what you need right before bed. When you exercise, your heart rate and blood pressure increase as well as your body temperature. While this may be great for energizing and increasing productivity during the day, this is not ideal for getting ready for bed.

I cannot emphasize enough that developing these good habits will benefit you in very concrete ways. But jumping into large changes, just like a fad diet or a New Year's resolution, has a tendency to be less successful. Take small, meaningful steps in the direction you set as an ultimate goal, and you will be much more likely to maintain them. The time before bed should be sacred. Use it wisely and develop a routine that you can stick to and you will notice that you have yet another tool in your belt to assist in preventing this potent migraine trigger.

Module 8: Preparing for Bed

I've been told by countless patients, and indeed have experienced myself, the way in which overthinking can become a problem. This is particularly frustrating when trying to fall asleep at night. Overthinking can easily be exacerbated by the technology that we have all become necessarily attached to. The TV, your phone, or other devices bombard you with information and drama that can undoubtedly get into your head. The goal of this module is to provide you with a tool to settle your unwanted thoughts, and prepare you for a smoother, more relaxed transition to bedtime. Feel free to engage in this now, or wait until you are planning to get ready for bed.

For this exercise, you will review your day, step-by-step, without judgment. This is not the time to dissect every interaction you had. You are merely observing as a bystander. Acknowledge the day's events and move on. It is perfectly fine if you want to lay down in bed for this module, but any position will do. Preferably done up to an hour before bedtime, this is meant to compose your mind to begin to quiet down and get ready for sleep. It has the additional benefit of improving your memory and strengthening recall. Take a moment and settle into whichever position you choose. Relax your eyes and adjust your body to be as comfortable as possible.

Take a nice, slow, deep breath. Begin with your morning. Recall the moment you awoke, still lying in bed, and before you got up. Think about how you felt after a night's sleep. Were you well rested? What time did you get up? Did you snooze your alarm? What clothing were you sleeping in? Did you have time for breakfast? If so, what did you eat? How did you get ready for your day? Did you shower or wash up? Did you have time to brush your teeth? What were you getting ready to do? Perhaps you had errands that you had to run?

Now, think about the day. This part is going to vary a lot from person to person, so take some time to pause here and think about it. You might want to go through it hour-by-hour. For example, where were you at 9 am? 10 am? And so on. Or section it by early versus late morning and early versus late afternoon.

It is quite natural for your mind to wander while you are doing this exercise. Simply take note of wherever your thoughts went, and acknowledge without any negativity, that you are "thinking" and return to observing the experiences of your day. Remember to retrace your steps in a non-judgmental manner, just acknowledging the course of events. Take your time. What did you eat today? Was it just snacking, or were you able to sit down for an actual meal?

Every time you find yourself drifting off and thinking of something else, or getting caught up in one particular moment, be kind to yourself. Acknowledge that you are thinking, and move back to the next recalled episode in your day. Now, move on to the early evening. If you were out, when did you get home? Did you have dinner? How did you spend your evening? Take the time to consider. Have you started to get ready for bed yet? At this point, you should be arriving at this present moment. If you need more time to review, take a minute to complete the process. Remember, just pass over each experience without perseverating on any. Merely observe and keep moving.

Before you continue, take a second to think about the next few steps required to get ready for bed. Whether it's showering, changing, or brushing your teeth, itemize these steps in your mind. Remember to limit phone and device use, as well as TV to an absolute minimum from now until you are asleep. Keep things quiet, calm, and relaxing. I wish you the most wonderful and restful sleep tonight.

CHAPTER 6:

Underlying
Medical Conditions

This chapter will focus on another general trigger of migraines, underlying medical diseases. Certain conditions may put you at higher risk for developing headaches, or experiencing migraines as part of another primary health issue. Regardless of the original cause, the final outcome in this case is a headache that needs management. Although the treatments for pain may be fairly similar, treating the root cause, whenever possible, is almost always going to be the best way to prevent and address the resulting discomfort.

Some of the most common conditions associated with increased risk of headache disorders include cardiovascular disease, neurologic syndromes such as epilepsy and sleep disorders, psychiatric disorders such as depression, anxiety, and PTSD, as well as other conditions like asthma and autoimmune disease (Burch et al, 2019). For people with diabetes, which can lead to widespread downstream systemic effects, poor long-term control of elevated sugar can cause many problems. Episodes of low blood sugar can also result in headaches

(Haghighi et al, 2016). Chronic pain syndromes including back pain and fibromyalgia are other common contributors to headache risk as well.

Fibromyalgia is a multidimensional diagnosis associated with extensive musculoskeletal pain and often accompanied by mood disorders, fatigue, and sleep disturbances. Note that these symptoms are also some of the most common migraine triggers that we discussed earlier. Patients often have chronic discomfort that is extremely difficult to manage and can be quite debilitating. It should not be surprising that these disorders can place patients at greater risk of developing headaches. Many people in these categories are already seeing pain management specialists and neurologists for assistance with their symptoms, and headaches in these patients are often an added insult to an already significant injury.

High blood pressure has been cited to me countless times as the cause of a patient's headache. While there was a historic belief in the medical community that there blood pressure can cause headaches, there does not appear to be strong evidence that it does so (Cortelli et al, 2004; Arca et al, 2019). Hypertension has been thought to contribute to headaches due to sudden increases in pressure. This may lead to localized swelling, bleeding, or lack of appropriate blood flow, which can result in pain (Arca et al, 2019). There are several situations during which we lower the blood pressure rapidly in the emergency department, such as aortic dissection, preeclampsia, and heart failure. In these cases there is a significant volume of research indicating a direct benefit to the patient by rapidly lowering their blood pressure. However, headaches associated with high blood pressure do not seem to improve in the emergency room even when blood pressure is rapidly controlled (Friedman et al, 2014).

Of course, a thorough exam is called for to rule out any danger-ous forms of headache in general, as we have discussed previously. Just like any other painful or anxiety-provoking condition, headaches may often cause a temporary increase in blood pressure (Peixoto, 2019). Often, when patients are in the throes of a painful migraine and nervous about its possible danger to them, their blood pressure is being pushed up from several angles. Both pain and anxiety are well-known causes of increased blood pressure. Many times, I find that just treating the pain from the headache alone, along with some gentle reassurance, will bring the blood pressure down to a more palatable number.

As noted earlier, strokes are one of the more dangerous types of headache presentations that we see in the emergency department. Post-stroke pain is a very important underlying medical condition in chronic headaches as well (Delpont et al, 2018). Nearly 50 percent of all stroke patients are affected by this (Hansen et al, 2012). Typically, these headaches resemble tension headaches, and they are often amenable to similar therapy.

In the introduction, I mentioned that women are affected by headache syndromes at about twice the rate that men are. There are some women who get migraines almost exclusively around the time of their menstrual period. This can occur for several reasons, including the fact that painful menstrual cramping can also cause stress which is a known factor that may contribute to headache pain and frequency. Another possibility is that there are fluctuations in hormonal balance, which can place some women at higher risk for headaches.

There are several hormonal systems that become more active at the onset of puberty. These produce higher amounts of hormones such as estrogen and testosterone as well as cortisol. These hormones have direct effects on the neurons in the brain, and regulation of the stress response. There is a lot of overlap to these systems, and they are involved in much more than just stress and sex, but we will focus on these effects for the purpose of our narrative. We already discussed the effects of stress, and its contributions to migraine, and knowing that it becomes more engaged at puberty may not come as much of a surprise. As the sex hormones become more active, their role in headaches does too. From the onset of puberty until menopause, women have more frequent fluctuations in these systems, and are at higher risk for headaches. Women who experience migraines are twice as likely to experience them with the onset of menses, and controlling the relative drop in estrogen levels has been found to improve symptoms. In fact, women who have "menstrual migraines" may often opt to take birth control pills in order to moderate hormonal fluctuation, hopefully leading to diminished migraines (Calhoun, 2018).

Birth control may not be an appropriate choice for everyone, of course. Some people have social, religious, or personal reasons for not wanting to or not being able to use hormonal birth control. Awareness alone that underlying medical factors can serve as potentiating triggers can still provide an advantage. By attending to and preventing a relatively predictable course, some relief can be obtained. This may mean making an effort to more carefully control your blood sugar if you have diabetes. Perhaps it is employing physical therapy for someone who has suffered a devastating injury or stroke. If you know that your headaches could be triggered by external factors, you can mentally prepare for this and prevent some of your symptoms by achieving a more optimal frame of mind. Mindfulness can be an effective instrument to improve your awareness (Creswell et al, 2016).

Module 9: Body Awareness

The goal of this module is to bring your attention to your body in a non-judgmental way. It should help increase your awareness of physical sensations and connect them to your emotions on a deeper and more centered level. While you can start at any part of the body and move in any direction, for this module, we will proceed from bottom to top. This is to guide your attention to how every part of your body leads up to your mind, and works together as an energy-building unit.

First, take a moment to find a comfortable position. Be mindful of all of the places that your body is in contact with the chair or whatever surface is beneath you. Relax your eyes and really allow yourself to settle into this space. Take a nice, slow, deep breath. We are going to establish an awareness of your entire body, starting with your feet and moving up to your head. Take another slow breath, and then allow your respirations to settle into your natural rhythm.

Now turn your attention to the bottoms of your feet. Are they pressed up against the ground? Or are they elevated? Are you wearing socks or shoes? Perhaps you are wearing slippers or sandals? Whatever is touching your feet right now, whether it's shoes, the floor, or even if it's only air, really pay attention to that sensation. Feel free to wiggle your toes a little if you can. Move your ankles a bit to get your feet moving up and down, right and left, and rotate if it feels comfortable for you to do so.

Now gently bring your attention just a little higher to your legs. Think about your lower extremities all the way from your ankles up to your hips. What are they feeling right now? How does the clothing that you are wearing feel against your skin? Give each leg a soft, gentle shake. Flex and extend your knees just a little. Now do the same with your hips. Really notice the feeling of your legs in this moment.

Now we are going to move up to your pelvis and stomach. Once again, focus on the sensation of your clothing or whatever surface is in contact with your skin. Shift around a little in your seat. Notice how every breath you take moves your stomach in and out. Take a moment to appreciate how your breathing activates motion all the way down to this level. What sensations do you notice here?

Now, move your attention further up to your chest and back. Keep following the way in which your breathing affects the expansion of your chest. In and out, along with every breath. How does this change the way your skin feels against your clothing? Straighten your back and expand your lungs. Notice how this position inherently makes you feel more confident, with your chest puffed out. Take another deep breath while focusing on your chest. Feel it rise and fall.

Now move on to your arms. Are you wearing long sleeves or are your arms bare? Are they resting on something, or hanging by your sides? There is no wrong answer, just be aware of the sensation of the material or of the air in contact with your skin. Move your hands and wiggle your fingers. Close your hand into a fist and give it a gentle squeeze. Notice how that affects your forearms. Flex and extend your elbows. Shake your arms out and rotate your shoulders just a bit. Now relax your hands and arms, and bring your focus up to your neck.

Soften the muscles around your neck and allow the tension to slip away. Range your neck by moving it slowly forward, then in a circular motion, up and around to the right. Then tilt back as you rotate towards the left, and finally bring it forward again. Now do the same in the opposite direction, slowly rotating it around. What do you feel there? Any warmth or coolness? Any soreness or ache?

Bring your attention to your face. Be aware of the muscles around your mouth as you smile. Now purse your lips like you are drinking through a straw, and hold it there for a few seconds. Then allow your mouth to relax. Move your attention to the area around your eyes. Squint just a little, and raise your eyebrows. Now allow all the muscles on your face to relax while you move your attention to your ears. Do you notice any tingling or warmth in that area? What do you feel on your scalp? Are you aware of any tingling or sensations there?

Now take this final moment to pay attention to your body as a whole. Take a nice deep breath and give yourself another little movement from top to bottom. How do you feel right now, in this moment? This is your body, and allowing yourself to appreciate it, will also be the tool that you need to become as healthy and as happy as you can be.

CHAPTER 7:
Sensory Triggers

While the triggers listed in the previous chapters are quite common, there are many others that are just as important for certain individuals. Some of these include environmental stressors, such as bad weather, loud sounds, bright lights, and strong smells. Specific foods or chemicals such as dairy, gluten, or chocolate, as well as chemicals including MSG, sulfites, and nitrites all may play a role in headaches.

While dairy has been cited to cause headaches in some unfortunate people, it is thought that the actual culprit may be a substance called tyramine. This food breakdown chemical can be found in products such as aged cheese, beer, and wine. While this has been studied at length, the exact mechanism for this relationship remains unclear. It is thought that alterations in dopamine levels or blood flow in the brain may play a role. However, it seems that not all tyramine containing products cause headaches, and multiple studies on the topic have come up with mixed results, thus bringing us back to the complexity of this disorder.

Chocolate, as a trigger, seems to have a very weak evidence base as well (Martin et al, 2016). It is important to note that chocolate contains a varying amount of caffeine as well. My mother has been obsessed with chocolate for as long as I can remember. She also suffered from migraines for many years, though the two never appeared to be causally related. So, if you are a chocoholic, you are probably ok to continue indulging. Everything in moderation of course.

Gluten is another cited trigger, and is found in foods such as wheat, grain, and barley. As celiac disease has become diagnosed more frequently, gluten has gained some renown as a possible culprit in other disorders as well. There is certainly an association of migraine symptoms in people diagnosed with celiac disease. These patients have an abnormal immune system response to gluten with the production of self-directed antibodies, and dietary control has been noted to improve their migraine symptoms. However, a gluten-free diet does not appear to help those that do not have celiac disease (Beuthin et al, 2020).

Monosodium glutamate, also known as MSG, is found in some foods such as tomatoes and cheese, and is often added to many processed goods for flavor. This is another commonly reported headache trigger. The mechanism may have to do with the binding of this chemical to certain receptors in the brain causing a disruption in blood flow. However, the available literature has not yet found a direct causational effect (Obayashi et al, 2016).

Nitrates and nitrites are used as food preservatives. Nitrates are found in cured meats and green, leafy vegetables such as spinach. Nitrates are converted to nitrites in the gastrointestinal tract, typically assisted by the normal bacterial flora that lives in the gut. They are thought to contribute to headaches, possibly by causing increased blood flow to the brain (Olesen et al, 2008). In fact, we often give nitroglycerin in the emergency department to patients complaining of chest pain. This is another nitrogen containing compound, and headaches are a well-described side-effect of this therapy, possibly related to the same impact on blood flow.

Sulfites occur naturally in wine, and are used as food preservatives as well. Though alcohol is a well-known migraine trigger in and of itself, it has been suggested that the sulfites contained in wine may make migraines worse for susceptible individuals. The actual mechanism for sulfite's role is unclear. However there has been some research indicating that perhaps high amounts of sulfites could affect headache development (Silva et al, 2019). Regardless of the food type or even the level of research currently available, if you notice a direct relationship between any food and your headaches, there is very little harm in attempting careful diet modification to see if you have any improvement.

In addition to foods, there are many other environmental causes of headache. As a general point, any change in the weather can potentially serve as a trigger (Li W. et al, 2019). Higher relative humidity and air pollution have been noted to have significant correlations. This can be due to electrical or neurochemical changes in the brain, or from a stress response to bad weather. For example, on hot days, we may forget to drink enough fluids. This could result in dehydration which can certainly provoke headaches. Or on gray days, we may be more subject to feelings of anxiety or depression, both well-known triggers. However, headaches can also occur as a direct reaction to the environment, and may involve barometric pressure changes in the atmosphere. There are multiple theories as to why this might be, and they include increased pressure or reduced blood flow in the brain, as well as increases in sinus pressure (Maini et al, 2019).

One of the more common and interesting triggers that my patients have presented with is strong smells. Some patients who experience this have been shown to have increased blood flow to areas associated with the olfactory system of the brain. This hyper-sensitivity to smells may activate the trigeminal system, which has been implicated in migraines (Bernardo et al, 2020). Such patients may be feeling fine, when suddenly they encounter a noxious odor. Shortly thereafter, they begin to notice symptoms of their migraine taking hold.

The same issue can occur with loud noises or bright lights. These are a few of the most commonly cited provoking factors. The real question about some of these things is whether or not they are triggers at all, or perhaps they are actually symptoms of migraine aura (Schulte et al, 2015). Many times, these symptoms are experienced hours before a migraine. I usually know when I am going to get hit by a migraine when everything around me seems louder than usual and I am in a pretty grouchy mood. However, it is difficult to distinguish sometimes whether it is part of your disease process or if it's actually causing it. While not always avoidable, having an awareness of your personal triggers is incredibly valuable in determining how you can set up your own environment to handle headaches. This is one of the reasons why keeping a headache journal is so important. We will discuss this in more detail later on.

Mold and allergies can be grouped together with asthma in an association of related conditions that can also function as triggers. They are connected via the concept of atopy. This is a genetic predisposition to be at risk for diseases like asthma, allergies, and certain skin conditions such as eczema. People suffering from these problems tend to have overactive immune responses to many environmental exposures like weather changes, mold, certain foods, and dust. Allergens are thought to be able to activate the trigeminal nerve system with increased inflammation (Bektas et al, 2017), making patients more prone to headaches.

The list of possible stressors is extensive. Not all of these will be causal in nature, but it is important to maintain a level-headed approach to evaluating each one as it pertains to you. While there may seem to be a myriad of triggers out there, keep in mind that addressing them individually with small, sustainable steps, can lead to important and lasting benefits in your life. The next few modules are aimed at utilizing your senses to increase awareness of your surroundings and your triggers. You may read them in the order listed, or individually at your leisure. The key is to provide yourself with as many tools as you can and find the ones that work for you.

Module 10: Aromatherapy

The capacity to detect smells is one of the most basic and primal senses that we possess. Your olfactory system is proficient at discerning the tiniest hint of chemical compounds in the air, and interpreting them with unimaginable precision. Smells have the power to change the way we perceive things and they have a strong impact on our sense of taste as well. As noted above, some people have certain smells that can trigger their migraines. This module will attempt to capitalize on the very same mechanism in order to fight them and to bring a sense of inner peace to your day.

Please find a nice, comfortable position. Take a moment to settle into the space that you chose. Relax your eyes and take a slow, deep breath. Breathe in through your nose and silently think to yourself, "In," and out through your mouth and think, "Out." Again, breathe in through your nose, thinking "In" and out through your mouth, thinking "Out." One more time, breathe in, thinking, "In," and breathe out, thinking, "Out."

Now relax your focus on your breathing and prepare to expand on the visualization skills that we have been practicing. Imagine yourself in the middle of a vast meadow. It is a pleasantly warm day and you are surrounded by a massive field of lush, green grass. In the distance you can hear some birds chirping and feel a gentle breeze, but otherwise, all is quiet. Looking around you, you see that this luxurious field has just been cut, and you can begin to smell that sweet, refreshing scent of freshly cut grass. Take a moment to imagine this smell.

Let this mellow but magnificent aroma caress your inner nares and breathe in slowly and deeply, filling your lungs with its perfume. Now, slowly let it out. Breathe again, in through your nose, and out through your mouth. Imagine yourself laying down on this thick, soft bed of greenness and allow that delicate freshness to bathe you in its warmth. Look closely at each blade of grass, and watch it glisten in the afternoon sun. Pick up a few pieces of the freshly cut grass in your hands and turn them over in your fingers. Take a moment here to really imagine what they might feel like in your hands.

Bring your face closer to the ground and take another deep breath, slowly. Allow the scent to travel through you and immerse you in its essence. Where is it taking you? What else does it make you think about? Does it remind you of pleasant memories from long ago? Listen to the gentle breeze as it moves the grass on the ground. Feel the warmth of the air around you as you enjoy this moment for just a few more seconds. Close your eyes for a moment to really imagine this.

Now begin to release your focus on this setting, and concentrate on breathing for a little while longer. Breathe in slowly. Breathe out slowly. Breathe in, and breathe out. Breathe in, and out.

Now you can let go of your focus on your breathing as well, and reflect on this exercise. The sense of smell is such a fundamental and primitive instinct, and it can bring you instantly to a whole new place and state of being. Allow it to be another tool for you in times of need. If you had a hard time imagining a smell, find an object that has a smell that you really love, and practice this technique again. Remember, there is no wrong way to do this. Just be kind and patient with yourself, and find a way that works for you.

Module 11: Sound Effect

As noted above, awareness can provide certain benefits, including giving the ability to recognize and treat provoking triggers that may be contributing to headaches. One of the most important rewards of increased awareness is better self-control which can further add to our capacity to address triggers. This works by managing bad habits and developing good ones as well. Awareness can also improve creativity, critical thinking in dealing with real-time situations, and increase your empathy towards other people. Though all of your senses are important in developing this skill, today, we will emphasize one in particular. By focusing your attention on the sounds around you, you will note a general improvement in your ability to listen in general, both to others, as well as to yourself.

Normally, a silent space is considered ideal for meditative purposes, and if this is what you choose, that is ok. For this exercise, it may be better to allow more of the outside world to filter in. Take a moment to find a comfortable location. Open the window or leave the door a little ajar if you can, so that some of the ambient noise from the environment can reach you. I recommend a seated, upright position, but as always, find something that works for you. Settle in, and sit with your chin held slightly upwards in a position of confidence. Relax your eyes. Take a slow, deep breath and be mindful of your body in this space. Straighten your back, and extend your neck just a little bit.

Soften your brow and your eyes, and unclench your jaw. Take note of your breathing as you gently inhale and exhale. Now, begin to pay attention to the sounds around you. You might hear noises from the street, like traffic. Or you may hear children laughing and playing. Perhaps you can hear birds chirping. You may notice sounds from inside as well, like people talking, or footsteps above you or in another room nearby. Maybe you notice the sounds the pipes are making in the walls. Listen to the heat or air conditioning, or the creak of a home settling. Even the sound of your own breath, as it flows in and out of your nose and mouth can be an interesting point of focus.

Notice these sounds without judgment. Simply listen to the natural symphony of the world around you at this moment, in this place. Ok, now you will pick one sound from around you and begin to hone in on this alone. There is no wrong sound to choose, and if the one you picked fades away or disappears, feel free to move on to another. Which sound called out to you? Is it light and high-pitched? Is it low and deep? Does it come and go? Is it regular or irregular? Is it loud, or very soft? The more detail you can identify about the sound, the more heightened your awareness of it will be.

You may notice that your mind has begun to wander while you are listening, and that is entirely ok and completely natural. Merely acknowledge that you are thinking, with the word, "thinking," and gently nudge your mind to return to find the sound you chose. Keep this focus for a little while longer, pause here for a minute or two to give yourself the space to appreciate what you are hearing.

Now let this sound drop back again among the other ambient noises around you. Once again, allow yourself to be immersed in the gentle symphony of the world where you are right at this moment. Exploring awareness is a great way to practice and build techniques in noticing our surroundings, or even changes in our own bodies. Take the time to pay attention, and you may find that you are building another mindfulness tool that can be applied in any way that you need.

Module 12: Out of Sight

For this module, we will continue our emphasis on increasing general awareness, this time utilizing sight. Remember, this capacity can provide you with the means to better identify your triggers, and hopefully serve to prevent migraines. We are often so preoccupied with our day-to-day lives that we forget to pay attention to the world around us. While this might serve a function by preventing us from getting caught up in minutia, it is this very attention to detail that is sometimes so important to focus on in order to brighten our perspective. This is a challenging module to read and perform at the same time, so I recommend that you read through first and then practice on your own.

Find a nice, quiet space to sit, preferably in an upright position. We will begin with eyes relaxed as usual, but soon, you will use your eyes to focus on your surroundings. Even if you are comfortable with meditation, it can be somewhat disconcerting to attempt it with your eyes open if you have never tried it before. Take your time and I am sure that you will find great value in exploring awareness with your vision.

With your eyes relaxed, settle into the space around you. Keep your chin a little elevated and relax the muscles around your eyes and face. Unclench your jaw. Take a nice, deep breath. Listen to your breath as it enters your nose, and again as you breathe it out through your mouth. Pay attention to any sounds that you hear around you.

Breathe in, and breathe out. Breathe in, and breathe out. Breathe in, and out. In, and out.

In a few moments, you will begin to focus your eyes. When you do, try not to focus on any one thing right away; just allow your eyes to settle on the general space in front of you. When you are ready, slowly direct your eyes to the area in front of you. Keep your gaze loose and intentionally out of focus. Notice what is there, but don't focus on anything in particular. Now try to see if there is one specific object that draws your attention and catches your eye. There is no wrong answer; it can be anything at all.

Let's examine the object you chose. What shape is it? Are its edges round? Or squared? What color is it? Does it have one color or many? Is it dark or light? How heavy is it? Really pay attention to all of the details of this object to increase your awareness.

It is entirely normal and ok if your thoughts have started to wander off during this exercise. Simply label this, "thinking," acknowledge your thoughts, and gently guide yourself back to focusing on the object of your choice.

Is this object large? Or small enough to hold in your hands? Does it have a rough surface? Or is it smooth?

Now, you may relax your gaze. Without looking again, try to picture the object that you chose. How many of the details can you envision in your mind? Feel free to release your focus now. Allow the thoughts and image of your object to fade away.

How did it feel to pay such close attention to an object? What was your experience like when you tried to picture it again without looking or with your eyes closed? Try to practice this skill when you have a moment and see if you can improve the image retention in your mind by paying more attention to the specific characteristics. Hopefully, as you build this skill, it will allow you to catch more of your triggers as well as improving your general awareness of the world around you.

CHAPTER 8:

Medications

M edications can be an enormous blessing and source of relief when it comes to headaches. Some of the most common over-the-counter formulations include drugs such as ibuprofen, acetaminophen, aspirin, and caffeine. There are many prescription options as well, geared towards addressing a number of the associated conditions related to headaches in general, and migraines in particular. Some are involved in prevention, or treating underlying conditions, and others address active headache symptoms. There are several neurochemicals and pathways in the brain that are thought to be involved in headaches. Here we will discuss some of the medications that are utilized to address them.

A few of the most commonly prescribed treatments for rapid symptom relief include the "triptan" family, such as sumatriptan and rizatriptan. I have personally experienced incredible improvement from both of these drugs. While mindfulness has really helped me in dealing with my own migraines, I am truly grateful for medication as well. It can make me feel a little drowsy after taking it, but it is a welcome change from the pain I was enduring. Triptans work primarily on the serotonin system to provide relief. Serotonin is a chemical produced by your body that is involved in many processes including mood stabilization and sexual desire. Controlling the levels of serotonin in the brain decreases inflammation and leads to a reduction in nerve-related pain.

In Chapter 1, we discussed the relationship between migraines and cluster headaches. One of the commonalities of the two involve a neurochemical called Calcitonin G-Related Peptide (CGRP). (Ljubisavljevic et al, 2018). CGRP is produced by neurons, and participates in communicating pain in the nervous system. It has been measured at high levels during migraines. In addition to controlling serotonin, triptan medications also ease migraines by blocking CGRP. More recently, a class of medications called gepants, including ubrogepant and rimegepant, has been developed specifically to target these peptides (Edvinsson et at, 2019).

Another chemical in the brain thought to be implicated in headache symptoms is dopamine. We know that dopamine plays a large role in the body by regulating muscle control and sexual desire, and it is heavily involved in the reward and reinforcement system. One of the most common medications we use in the emergency department for migraine relief is metoclopramide. Medications in this class are thought to help by blocking dopamine receptors, leading to decreased levels in the brain (Khazazi et al, 2019). They block another chemical called histamine as well, resulting in reduced nausea and vomiting. This is particularly useful in many migraine attacks. One of my favorite medications to use in particularly resistant headaches is haloperidol. This drug also works primarily on the dopamine pathway with antihistamine effects. While it tends to be very effective, it is unfortunately relegated to a backup option since it also interacts with many other receptors in the brain, causing it to have a higher risk of side effects.

Another less commonly utilized type of migraine treatment includes the ergot alkaloids. This class of medication includes dihydroergotamine and ergotamine and mainly works by interacting with serotonin receptors (Shafqat et al, 2020). The reason these are rarely used in clinical practice is the significant side effect profile that includes increased cardiovascular risk, abdominal pain, nausea, and vomiting. However, these may still be employed in very select cases for particularly resistant headache syndromes.

I would be remiss if I didn't discuss the implication of opioids and opiates in the management of headaches. Drugs in this category include morphine, hydromorphone, and fentanyl among others. They act by binding to opioid pain receptors in the central nervous system which blocks the perception and response to pain (Choi, 2016). While there is no doubt they are powerful and rapidly effective painkillers, they have a tendency to induce sensitization, increasing the risk of medication overuse headaches, and may diminish the effectiveness of other medications as well (Ong et al, 2018). This means that while they might work to rapidly decrease pain in the moment, they have a tendency to make patients more sensitive to pain in the future, and make that pain more difficult to treat. These highly addictive medications have some very dangerous side-effects as well, including drowsiness, breathing problems, and death. Opiates have a long history of abuse, and there is a huge social cost related to that. Needless to say, I am not a fan of this approach.

Many classes of medications are employed that act on multiple pathways including anti-inflammatories as well as medications that work on the nervous system, all in the hopes of achieving some respite. Again, because of the complex nature of pain and the many theorized causes and triggers, it is not always clear what the best course of action will be. If these medications are required routinely, you and your doctor may opt to take a preventative migraine medication. There are many of these available, including pills, injectables, and more, and I would strongly encourage you to have a discussion with your doctor if you fall into this category.

It can be very tempting to jump to medications at the first instance of pain. Perhaps you are the kind of person who gets an aura prior to having a migraine. You may begin to experience some heightened sensitivity to light or sound, or you may notice squiggly lines in your field of vision. Whatever your aura is, you know that soon there is a good chance you will develop a migraine headache. It can certainly be alluring to take something that can provide some relief as early as possible. However, over time, many of these medications can come with unwanted side effects. Even ibuprofen and acetaminophen, among the most common components of headache regimens, can have a serious rebound effect when taken too often. This is similar in a sense to overeating or drug abuse. Your body gets used to these substances being present on a daily basis, and when they are suddenly taken away, you will feel very poorly in response.

If medications are only needed occasionally, this problem does not tend to arise, but if you suffer from very frequent headaches, then you are more prone to this. It is quite easy to develop these habits, because all you want is a little relief. That is completely rational. As time goes on, you may find yourself taking these medications earlier and earlier for your headaches as you develop a more keen sense of when they are going to occur. Increasingly, you may realize that if you try not to take medication for pain, you cannot even go one day without getting a headache. This is called a rebound headache, and the syndrome associated with it is called medication overuse headaches.

Medication overuse is defined by the International Classification of Headache Disorders (ICHD-3) as rebound headaches that occur in people with primary headache disorders associated with greater than 15 days of symptoms per month requiring medications on at least 10 – 15 of those days (Wakerly et al, 2019). These can be even more frustrating and challenging to treat than your original headaches because the normal therapies that you have come to depend on have now become a source of headaches themselves. So what can you do if your treatment has become a trigger? At this point, many patients and providers will opt for a preventative medication. There are several options which work on different pathways to achieve this goal.

These include medications that control blood pressure, like beta blockers and calcium channel blockers. These are thought to help by moderating the rate of blood flow and pressure changes to the brain. Anti-seizure medications such as topiramate or divalproex sodium are often used. The thought process behind this is that these medications may calm overactive nerves in the brain which may play a role in headaches. Antidepressants can help as well, especially for those with depression and anxiety as underlying triggers. Amitriptyline and Venlafaxine are among the most common antidepressants utilized in this way.

There are many preventative therapies that you can try, with more being developed all the time. Of course, along with the supervision of your doctor, there is great value to pursuing this if needed.

For the time being, I strongly encourage you to keep directing your mental resources towards treating all of the underlying triggers that you can. The next mindfulness module will use our perceptions of medication-induced relief as a form of treatment in and of itself.

Module 13: Take a Pill

The mind is an incredibly powerful resource. The manner in which you perceive the world around you can dramatically affect your experience. You have likely heard of the placebo effect. A classic example is when the effects of a new drug are being studied. Group A gets the experimental drug, and group B gets a sugar pill – the placebo. What is strange about the results of many of these studies is that even the placebo group seems to experience a noticeable effect, despite the fact that all they had was a sugar pill. Why would that be? This is a demonstration of the power of sugges-tion on the brain. If you really believe that something is going to affect you in a certain way, your mind manages to achieve some measurable change. What that tells us is that if we can harness that strength purposefully, we may be able to access a measure of the improvements that come along with the medications prescribed for headaches, but without the bothersome side effects. No matter where you are, or what time of day it is, you always have access to this particular asset.

Take a moment to find a comfortable space for your body. If you can dim the lights, or go somewhere quiet, even better, but any position in any location will do. Relax your eyes and settle in. Take a deep, slow breath.

Breathe in, and breathe out. Breathe in, and breathe out. Breathe in, and out. In, and out.

We are now going to use our imaginations again, in the hopes of providing some real relief with the power of visualization. Bring to mind the image of a pill bottle, the kind you might get when picking up a prescription in the pharmacy. Lift it up in your mind, and give the bottle a light shake. You will hear the sound of one solitary pill rolling around within. Untwist the cover and look inside. There is a pill sitting at the bottom of this bottle. The color, shape and size are up to you. Take a moment before continuing to envision this pill.

What color did you think of? Is it more of a dull shade, or bright neon? What shape is it? A perfect circle like a tablet? Perhaps it has one of those lines down the center, to make it easier to cut? Or is it oval-shaped like a capsule? Now think of the size of the pill. How big is it? Super small, like a baby-aspirin? Or extra-large? Or maybe somewhere in between?

Whichever way you decided, focus on this pill and make it your own. Turn it around in your mind and examine it from all sides. How does it reflect the light? What does it feel like to the touch? How would it feel to put it into your mouth? Imagine it on your tongue. Does it feel dry? Is it rough, or is it smooth? Imagine that as you sit with this pill in your mouth, you begin to salivate. You notice that the pill has begun to dissolve on your tongue. You feel the urge to swallow. Now, imagine a cool glass of water sitting on a table to your side. It glistens with moisture on its surface and it looks fresh and clean.

You pick up the glass and bring it to your lips. The water passes into your mouth and the gently dissolving pill is swept off your tongue and heads to the back of your throat as you swallow. This pill is filled with a powdery mysterious tonic. Already, your body begins to break down the pill and its magic begins to seep into your body. Microscopic molecules of relief come bustling out and join your bloodstream, being carried rapidly to all areas of your pain. You feel relief radiating to your shoulders and neck, then to your jaw and face, and up to your eyes and forehead. You feel the effects all the way to the top of your scalp. There is a soft, tingling respite everywhere it goes, bathing you in gentle light and relief. You imagine a glow about you as your pain washes away.

Enjoy this experience for a moment longer. Just relax and acknowledge whatever you are feeling right now. Take a nice, slow, deep breath. Feel all of the muscles loosen around your shoulders, neck, face, and jaw. Pay special attention to the area behind your eyes and the top of your head. All of these locations are releasing their tension and softening their muscles. Now you may begin to let go of the focus you had on this exercise.

I hope that you were able to find a modicum of support with this segment and perhaps it can help you develop the tools you need to prevent the cycles of discomfort we experience. You may have noticed that this module may did not fit precisely into the mindfulness category, but was rather more like self-directed hypnosis and an exercise of the mind. That is ok. The important factor here is finding multiple modalities to treat and prevent pain. Finding the avenue that works for you may be just as multifaceted as headaches themselves. Please feel free to come back to this module or any other as often as you like and try to make use of all of your senses to envision a little relief.

Chapter 9:
Diet

I am often asked by patients what foods they can eat to help with various conditions. Nausea, vomiting, diarrhea, and abdominal pain are all intuitive symptoms where diet can play a role, and diagnoses like diabetes and high blood pressure can certainly be at least partially managed with diet control. However, there are many other medical conditions with which nutritional monitoring can assist. There is no specific type of food or drink that will completely alleviate headaches. But keeping a generally healthy and balanced diet will contribute to overall wellbeing and that alone can play a large role in diminishing triggers.

First, let's break down food into its vital components. There are carbohydrates, fats, proteins, vitamins, and electrolytes. Most foods contain more than one, and often several, of these elements. Without going into excessive detail, we will discuss some of their major characteristics. The two main types of carbohydrates can be divided into complex carbs and simple sugars. Complex carbohydrates are starches and include foods like bread, pasta, rice, and potatoes. Simple sugars are found in some of our greatest temptations such as candy, chocolate, and even fruits and vegetables. Fats come in all shapes and sizes, and some are absolutely vital for our health, giving us energy and the ability to metabolize certain kinds of vitamins. Fats are categorized as saturated, monounsaturated, polyunsaturated, and trans fats.

Unsaturated fats have been shown to increase the levels of LDL, one of the "bad" kinds of cholesterol, and are relatively difficult for the body to break down. Butter is a classic example of an unsaturated fat. You can almost imagine how large volumes of the creamy stuff can cause all sorts of damage to your arteries. Monounsaturated fat and polyunsaturated fats may actually decrease the levels of LDL, and are easier for the body to break down (Sacks et al, 2017). Monounsaturated fats are found in larger proportions in foods such as olive oil and avocados, while polyunsaturated fats can be found in fish, meat, and nuts. Trans fats are probably the most detrimental for your digestive system. Largely engineered by humans, though they exist in small amounts naturally in some foods, they are formed by the process of hydrogenation. This is most often observed in deep-fried fast foods, pastries, and some vegetable oils. Undoubtedly, they are delicious, but trans fats take a heavy toll on your body. This can lead to weight gain and metabolic syndrome, leaving you at much higher risk for things like heart attacks or strokes (Islam et al, 2019). When purchasing an item that boldly advertises that it is fat-free, but contains a ton of sugar, you are not doing your body any favors. In reasonable portions, fats that are not saturated or trans fats are actually important for overall health.

Proteins have extensive responsibilities in the body, and are involved in processes such as digestion, oxygen transportation and utilization, muscle growth, and strengthening of the immune system. Some of the more common sources of protein include meat, fish, eggs, nuts, and soy. They are an absolutely vital part of any well-balanced diet. Some diets, like veganism, can place you at risk for protein deficiency. This can be remedied by paying careful attention to intake from plant-based sources of protein such as greens like broccoli or kale, nuts and legumes, seitan, whole grains, and tofu.

There are many types of essential vitamins and electrolytes, and they are all important in various body functions and needs. I won't go through them all, but I will point out some common examples along with their key functions. Vitamin A is involved in eye and skin health and plays a supportive role in red blood cell development and the immune system. There are multiple types of vitamin B, and these function in many areas such as immune strength, preventing anemia, and promoting metabolism. Vitamin B6 and B12 are active in many of your body's cellular reactions, metabolism, and energy. Vitamin C has a number of different benefits, including development and maintenance of your musculoskeletal system, and is known to be involved in promoting healthy immunity. Vitamin D assists with these systems as well, and is particularly valuable in bone strength. This can be achieved with a little sunlight, but often, especially for those in colder climates, supplements are needed.

Free radicals can come from things like pollution, cigarette smoke, and certain products of digestion. Both Vitamin C and E are antioxidants, which help the body get rid of free radicals. Folate, also known as folic acid, is involved in blood cell production and is particularly important in pregnancy for healthy prenatal care. Vitamin K is noted for its involvement in blood clotting factors. The list of vital functions for vitamins is quite extensive, and like proteins, they are extremely important to overall well-being.

Electrolytes are essential minerals such as sodium, chloride, calcium, magnesium, and potassium. Each of these has a normal level in the human body, and remains balanced when you are in good health. Sodium and chloride are key players in cellular health and hydration. Calcium is well known for its role in strengthening bones and teeth. Iron is of special significance in blood cell production and preventing anemia. Potassium is involved in many areas including muscle contraction, nerve communication, and blood pressure control. Zinc plays a role in the immune system, helps support healthy skin, and contributes to your senses of smell and taste. There is often temptation to take large amounts of vitamins such a zinc or Vitamin C, especially for goals of disease prevention. The available literature does not support its use in this way, though they are typically safe to take in moderate doses. However, one must be cautious not to use in high doses for prolonged periods, because even vitamins can be detrimental when taken excessively.

Some nutrients have been touted specifically for their roles in migraine therapy. Magnesium in particular has been studied extensively for migraine prevention and treatment. The effects are likely minimal, but in small doses, it is also quite safe. Magnesium is also known for its properties of cardiac and nerve stabilization. Vitamin B2, also known as riboflavin, has been cited as a possible migraine deterrent. Coenzyme Q-10 is a nutrient involved in cardiovascular health that works as an antioxidant, and is thought to help with migraine prevention as well. Butterbur, an herb made from the leaves of the shrub with the same name, may have value when it comes to migraine avoidance. While it could have some moderate effects, don't expect anything too magical. If you think you may benefit from these supplements, I encourage you to speak to your doctor or headache specialist.

Electrolyte balance is the one area which is most actively involved when dealing with severe headaches. It needs to be closely monitored. When you are not feeling well, whether from a headache or any other ailment, your appetite may not be as hearty as usual. If this only affects food ingestion, then this should not have any immediate impact on your electrolytes. However, if you are not drinking enough, then you are at risk for dehydration. Water is great, but fluids containing electrolytes such as Pedialyte or electrolyte-enhanced sports drinks are even better for this purpose. Dehydration can exacerbate your headache, creating a very vicious, and sometimes dangerous cycle. With migraines, this is often compounded with nausea and vomiting, which puts you at even greater risk.

As a preventative measure, it is always important to maintain proper hydration. This will ensure that you are not adding dehydration to the long list of triggers you may have. When you feel like you have a headache, please make it a point to work as hard as you can to avoid this issue, even if you don't have an appetite. This is one of the things that I see most in the emergency department. Often, after a small amount of fluid administration, a terrible headache can become much more manageable.

Addressing headaches when they occur is very important, but some of our eating behaviors can have negative consequences on a chronic level. Many people have a tendency to overeat, while others appear to have an easier time with self-control. It is vital to remember that there are many factors that contribute to these urges. How do we control ourselves when we have a desire to eat too much or to eat something we know we shouldn't? This is not the time to point out the inherent problems with overeating or with poor choices, like eating large amounts of candy. You already know these things. Now is the time to address the mental and emotional reasons for why we make these choices despite knowing better.

Treating these issues like an addiction will help you realize why and how they need to be addressed. When it comes to addiction, your mind has an amazing capacity to convince you to do something even if you know you shouldn't. The reward system in our brain is geared to respond to these stimuli and push your body to get more. This had tremendous value from an evolutionary perspective, because the body needs energy to survive. But before the advent of land cultivation and farming, there wasn't the overabundance of processed junk food that is available today. So the system is still in place in our minds, thanks to our ancient ancestors, but is now likely doing more harm than good.

It is important to note that many psychosocial factors play a role here as well. Access to healthy and affordable options may be somewhat limited, especially in less affluent communities. Culture is also a crucial factor to consider. If you grow up in an environment where the people around you all eat and live a certain way, whether or not it is healthy may be less important than fitting in to your society. There is a psychological element as well. Many people will readily admit that they are burying their feelings of depression and anxiety in food. Unfortunately, this is not the healthiest of mentalities, and will often lead to further burdens of metabolic syndrome, obesity, and poor cardiovascular health. These ailments can also be detrimental to your emotional wellbeing.

There is way too much available information regarding dietary recommendations, much of it conflicting. This can make it even more confusing when trying to determine what to eat, when to eat it, and how much of it to eat. Finding a good system of nutritional consumption, along with a well-balanced diet that is relatively low in trans-fats and saturated fats is the best advice I can give about how to maintain a healthy lifestyle. Try to have a little less salty and processed foods, and avoid candy and other sugary products like soda when possible. Availability and ease of access play a big role in eating choices. So, perhaps try packing some cut up carrots or celery when you are going to work. Replace that bag of chips with some unsalted, mixed nuts. If you have your lunch prepared in advance, then there will be less temptation to order from a local fast food restaurant. Combined with generally good habits, like sleep hygiene and physical fitness, this can lead to improved symptoms, decreased migraines, and overall better health. Of course, not everyone will be able to make these changes, and there are many reasons why this might be. Some things are not in your control, but do the best you can to work with what you have to make the most of your personal situation. And once again – small steps equal large changes.

Module 14: Diet Control

This module is meant to provide some insight into how we feel about food. That said, it can also be applied to other unwanted habits, such as smoking, or biting your fingernails. Feel free to apply these ideas to whichever negative urges are pertinent to you while utilizing this module.

When the sensation of hunger or other desires arise, it can be very tempting to immediately satisfy that urge. But remember, these triggers have a neurochemical basis. Our drive is based on a complex interaction that includes hormones and our rewards center. This actually only lasts briefly, because it is not energy-efficient for our bodies and minds to maintain that kind of focus for a prolonged period of time. There is only a short interval that the sensation is there, and if not immediately addressed, it fades into the background. Therefore, the tool you need does not have to completely inhibit these urges forever, just for a fleeting moment. This module is only meant to address negative habits, such as overeating. It is not meant to avoid normal feelings of hunger or to encourage you to skip meals completely. Keeping that in mind will help this to be a more readily attainable skill.

Take a moment to find a comfortable position, preferably sitting up. Relax your eyes, and settle into the space around you. If you are feeling the urge to overeat now, then this is a perfect opportunity to practice, and if not, keep these thoughts in mind when you are. It may be even more helpful to learn a new skill when you are at an optimal frame of mind. This will make it easier to apply when you are being put to the test. Straighten your back and neck, and elevate your chin a little. Take a slow, deep breath. Notice the way it makes your abdomen expand when you take a breath in, and how it settles when you breathe out.

If you can, place one or both of your hands on your stomach and feel the way this movement follows the pattern of your breathing. Breathe in, and your abdomen expands, and breathe out, it settles back down. Breathe in, and breathe out. Breathe in, and breathe out.

What is it that makes you want to eat right now? Is it an appropriate mealtime? Or are you in between meals and eating out of habit? Is it just seeing food that is out that makes you want it? Or will you have to go and obtain it first? Remember that when these urges are inappropriate, then the sensations will come in waves, and will only last for a short moment. When you are actually hungry for a meal, you will continue to be hungry until you eat. Think about this sensation now, and acknowledge that this feeling too, shall pass.

Take this opportunity to check in with yourself, and see if this is a time that you should actually eat, or if this food item is an appropriate choice. If not, note to yourself that this is just a passing wave. It will come, and then it will go. Your first inclination may be to say, yes, this is appropriate and I want it now. And that is normal. Your brain will attempt to validate your desires at any cost. But give this another moment, and ask yourself again. Is this the time to eat? If it is, is this an appropriate choice?

Wait a few seconds before answering again. You might find that now that you have given your brain permission to pause, to note that there may be an alternative drive, you can acknowledge that you might not actually be hungry. Perhaps there is another reason for you to want this food. Maybe it's because it is in front of you. Someone else is eating nearby? Maybe you are bored? Or do you habitually eat when doing a specific activity, like driving or watching TV?

No matter the outcome, give yourself a minute before moving on. Just settle again into the space around you and take a deep breath. Take a moment to appreciate the effort that you are making. The longer you pause to ask this question and wait an ample amount of time to answer, you may find that the wave has already begun to pass. If it has not, remember to try to make healthy choices, and of course you should eat when it is appropriate to do so. Use this tool as often as you need, and when paired with other methods of creating good habits, you'll find that these small, but meaningful steps will lead to lasting changes in your life.

Chapter 10:

Exercise

Physical fitness is especially important to your overall health and happiness, and can even be helpful in alleviating migraines (Amin et al, 2018). Of course, lifting weights or running on the treadmill is not curative by any means, and when you are actively in the throes of a miserable headache, it may be one of the last things you would consider doing. Unfortunately, sometimes physical exertion can be a trigger too, but as a preventative measure, exercise can increase blood flow to all parts of your body including your brain (Irby et al, 2015). It can improve your metabolism, your self-esteem, and bolster immunity, as well as overall physical and emotional health.

Beginning with your cardiovascular and pulmonary systems, exercise promotes increased oxygen use by all parts of your body. The more regularly you physically train, the more adept it is at tolerating various stressors. The first time you go for a run, you may note that you are short of breath after less than a minute. You may not have thought that you were out of shape, but when you stress your body in a new way, you might discover some unpleasant truths. However, if you continue to push yourself, your body will adapt to the challenge. This is true for weight training as well. The more you persist, the more weight you will be able to lift, or the more repetitions you will be able to perform. This also has the more subtle benefit of strengthening your blood vessels, potentially decreasing your risk of high cholesterol, heart attacks, and strokes.

While you are in the process of becoming more fit, you also tend to have an increased metabolism. This is certainly true while you are actively exercising, but metabolism seems to remain elevated for some time after as well (Knab et al, 2011). So, while you are sitting at your desk at work, or even vegging out in front of the TV later on, your body is still burning calories on a cellular level! Your body becomes more sensitive to insulin, which is involved in getting rid of excess sugar, minimizing your likelihood of developing conditions like diabetes, obesity, and metabolic syndrome (Bird et al, 2017). In addition to immediate changes like increased blood flow, the body can develop sustained improvements from exercise as well. Decreased cholesterol, anti-inflammatory effects, decreased cortisol, psychological health, and improved immunity are all well-described benefits (Li G. et al, 2020).

There are an abundance of exercise options available, including weight-lifting, cross-training, yoga, high-intensity interval training, and much, much more. Though there is a broad overlap, the most basic way to break down exercise is into two main categories; aerobic and strength training. Both of these types of exercises can be performed simultaneously, and often include subcategories of fitness like balance and flexibility. Directly addressing balance problems through exercise and physical therapy has been suggested as possible migraine therapy. However, the role of balance training in headache management remains more theoretical, as current evidence is lacking in terms of its purported benefits (Carvalho et al, 2019).

Aerobic exercise is more focused on increasing stamina and includes activities such as running, swimming, and biking. Often, the goals of these exercises are to get your heart moving harder and faster, and geared towards maximizing endurance. There have been several studies dedicated to evaluating aerobic exercise as a means to diminish migraine symptoms and effects, and there is some moderate evidence to support this (Lemmens et al, 2019). Strength training typically focuses on building muscle, and often utilizes techniques such as weight or resistance training. The focus of these types of activity is more on muscle tone, development, and mass. While there is evidence that increased intensity can have a greater benefit, even lower intensity exercise has been shown to help prevent migraines (Barber et al, 2020). This does not specifically differentiate between strength training and aerobics, but compares the level of intensity involved. Unfortunately, the data is somewhat limited in its quality and scope, and more research is needed on this topic before we can make any definitive recommendations (Lemmens et al, 2019).

There are many studies comparing the types of exercise on outcomes such as diabetes and metabolic syndromes, but overall, there is no strong evidence at this point to recommend one type over another (Nery et al, 2017). So, how are you to know which one is best for you and which method will prevent the most migraines? Unfortunately, this answer is likely going to vary from person to person, and will depend on a number of different factors. Age, gender, current level of physical conditioning, and chronic health problems and disabilities all may affect how or what kind of activity you can do.

The most important concept is to safely engage in exercise and progress as slowly as you need to. So if you haven't been off your couch in a few months, running a marathon tomorrow might not be the best idea. You are more likely to get hurt than get into shape that way. For some people, taking a short walk at a slow pace may be all they are capable of. If you are just starting out, small decisions like taking the stairs when you can, or parking a little farther from your destination can force you to exercise a little more. Regardless of your foundation, make the decision to start. Today. Create a plan to continue putting in effort without causing pain or placing yourself in danger. If you are not sure what you are able to do, I encourage you to seek professional guidance on how to safely get started and move forward. Even thinking about this right now is putting your mind in a better place. Once again, small steps lead to big and lasting changes.

Module 15: Energy Boost

This is a short, but powerful piece of mindfulness. Sometimes, you may have the right thoughts and interest in taking action, but you can't seem to actually motivate yourself to get started. This is particularly pertinent to exercise goals. Often, it is just about recruiting the energy that you need to begin. Once activated, your body's own adrenalin will keep you moving and you can ride that until you reach your goal. For now, we will aim to harness some of that energy through your breathing to jumpstart this system. We will utilize a technique known as breath of fire which comes from Kundalini yoga. If at any point you feel lightheaded or short of breath, please pause and return to your natural pace of breathing.

Find a comfortable position, preferably sitting upright with your back and neck straight. Relax your eyes. Bring your chest forward and elevate your jaw to a position of confidence. Raise your shoulders just a bit, and move your elbows a little away from your body if possible. Move your hands over your stomach, and breathe in deeply. Notice the air expanding your chest and abdomen. Really try to feel that power as you breathe it back out.

Now, you will take the next few breaths rapidly in and out through your nose. If you find it easier to breathe out through your mouth, that is ok as well. So, one more regular deep breath in, and now let it out slowly. Over about 10 seconds, you will breathe rapidly in and out through your nose. You should be able to get at least 20 breaths in and out.

Let's get started with the first round. Rapidly breathe in and out, hard and fast, through the nose. Try to keep this going for at least 10 seconds, or count at least 20 exhaled breaths.

If that made you lightheaded, slow your pace, or only take a few breaths. Take a nice, relaxed breath, in and out, and we will go on to the next round.

Round 2, rapidly breathe in and out, hard and fast, through the nose for at least another 10 seconds. Great, keep up the good work, and take another relaxed breath to recuperate. Feel that energy building.

Ok, round 3, rapidly breathe in and out, hard and fast, through the nose for at least another 10 seconds.

Fabulous. Now allow your breathing to return to your natural rhythm. Take a moment to rest before moving on to your next activity. I hope that you now have the energy you need for exercise or whatever other goals you have. Take advantage of the momentum you have started to build. Come back and utilize this technique as often as you like to give yourself a little extra boost whenever you need it most.

CHAPTER 11:

Perspective

O ften, especially with migraines that go on for days, it can seem like we are in a never-ending world of suffering. One of the best ways to keep things in perspective, while also assisting in identifying various triggers, is to keep a headache journal. The more detail you include, the more accurate a representation of the frequency and severity of your symptoms. Why is this important? By recognizing the particulars surrounding your headaches, you can pick out more of your personal triggers and address them individually. It can certainly be helpful to know that in the month of November, you had three more headaches than you had in October. But it would provide even more practical information if you add specific features about those events. What time of day did the headache occur? How long did it last? On a scale of one to ten, how bad was it? What interventions or medications did you try? How successful were they? What were the surrounding circumstances? This may be a little time consuming, but including characteristics like the weather, your level of stress, and your diet and exercise from those days, all can be helpful in narrowing down your own individual migraine stressors. This initial time investment will pay for itself in dividends of headache-free time that you can use in any way that you wish.

In addition to contributing to your general awareness, there is also an emotionally reassuring purpose to this practice. It can be comforting to be able to objectively quantify how much relatively symptom-free time we already have. It can serve as a reminder that not every single day is filled with distress. Being able to see this provides a level of hope, even when we are at our lowest. Recognizing the positive value in our lives enables us to achieve the optimism we need to manage the more difficult challenges we face.

There are many ways in which we can institute change in our lives. However, it can be very hard to maintain those changes once we start. There are a few techniques that I utilize to make my habit-forming goals a reality. The first is a method called pairing. This is accomplished by taking a daily routine, like brushing your teeth or making yourself a cup of coffee in the morning, and pairing it with another good habit that you want to develop. For example, every time you brush your teeth, you can also practice a short mindfulness module. Or you can do calf-raises. Or every time you make a cup of coffee, do a few pushups while waiting for the coffee to brew. You will find that the more often you pair the same activity with one you already do, the greater the likelihood of developing the good habit you're aiming for.

The second method utilizes your phone. Sure, our phones often get a bad rap as a source of attention-seeking, mind numbing proliferation of media, and rightfully so. But no one would argue that our phones are amazing devices. The sheer volume of functions, tools, and educational capacity of your phone is truly spectacular. This method is a simple one requiring only your calendar. Using this function for important birthdays or to schedule meetings is a great way to remember important events, but take it one step further. Schedule the habit that you want, preferably as a daily reminder. For example, put in a time for exercise. Or to study a language, or even just set a time to take a five-minute break for yourself. When you see it in writing, it can carry so much more weight than our usual resolutions that always seem to get forgotten somewhere along the way.

Another method I find very useful is setting small goals. This can be especially helpful when the task at hand is daunting, and the light at the end of the tunnel is nearly impossible to see. One of my favorite examples of this is a long race, like a marathon. You may not be able to see the finish line, and that has the potential to diminish your stamina, but you can see the person in front of you. So focus on that person until you pass them, and then focus on the next one. I use a similar technique on the treadmill. This is an activity I find particularly boring, but I know I will appreciate it after I'm done. So, I break down every session into individual minutes. I challenge myself only to focus on sixty seconds at a time. How fast can I run this minute? And before I know it, I have completed the exercise. I also apply this process to my workday. Thinking about a nine- or twelve-hour shift can seem formidable. So, I break it up into segments as well. I will have a coffee at the three-hour mark, a break to eat half-way, and maybe a tea at the six-hour mark. These can change based on my needs, and in the emergency department, my breaks aren't always at exact times, but the general idea is there. It makes the day much more manageable by focusing only on small bits of information, so that it is not overwhelming.

So, how do we go from our daily existence, with all of its built-in stressors, to a point of tranquility? The most important thing is to recognize what is causing that stress and keeping it in perspective. I heard a great analogy once from a teacher I had many years ago. In addition to possessing an amazing Cheech and Chong impression, he was always full of wise words and sage advice. During a particularly stressful time in my life, he pulled me to the side of the classroom to discuss some of my issues. After careful consideration, he told me to imagine a merry-go-round or carousel device, the type on which a child sits and grabs onto a wheel in the center to spin around. The faster the child turns the wheel, the faster they will spin. The key here is that the wheel is actually not moving at all. It is completely stationary. It is the child, sitting on the spinning platform that is moving around the wheel. The point is that the situation or stressor you are dealing with now is not necessarily the thing that needs to be moved. In fact, often it cannot be moved at all. Sometimes, the solution that you need is not achieved by moving the problem itself, but changing your own position to see things from another angle.

Module 16: A Distant Perspective

The next few mindfulness modules at the end of the book are geared towards providing you with improved perspective and emotional well-being. Please utilize them in any order that works for you. This one will focus on providing you with a tool to manage your headaches and triggers, again using the power of your imagination. You will envision yourself from the outside, creating an alternative perspective that you can come back to anytime with the hopes that it will achieve some symptom improvement.

Just like the carousel example above, sometimes the movement you need to bring about change is already within you.

Take a moment to find a comfortable space. There is no wrong position for you to be in. You can be sitting up in a position of confidence, reclining, or if you need to, feel free to lie down. Relax your eyes. Take a nice, deep breath, and slowly release it. Concentrate for just a moment on relaxing the muscles of your face, jaw, neck, and the area around your eyes.

We are now going to put your imagination to work. Think of this as an activity to strengthen your mind to better fight stress in much the same way physical exercise strengthens your muscles. First, you will think of something that is causing you stress right now. There is no wrong answer or choice here. It could be your job, a difficult co-worker, a fight with a loved one, economic hardship, or something more focal and specific, like having a headache or dealing with chronic pain. This tool can be applied to almost any scenario, so the first thing you think of is probably ok to focus on, especially knowing you can come back to this exercise as often as you like to address any stressor of your choice.

Now that you have chosen your stressor, we are ready to push your imagination. Continue to consider your stressor, no matter what it is, and imagine that you are no longer sitting or lying down in whatever area you are physically located right now. Rather, you are floating above your body, observing, but not feeling anything. You are still aware of the stressor, but now you are outside of it. You know that it is nearby, but it cannot touch you. Begin to zoom out, just a little, like on a digital map, still able to observe, but even farther away. You can still see yourself in the distance, but so much smaller. You can look around and notice many homes and buildings, parks, and perhaps a large body of water. You know your stressor is still right there, but you are barely able to perceive it.

You are now ready to zoom out again. You are floating high in the sky, gently caressed by white, pillow-like clouds while you look down on your distant self. You can see landscapes and large bodies of water, but no longer identify individual homes. The stressor still sits with your tiny body where you left it, but cannot follow you here. Zoom out again until you are perched up among the stars. Looking down at the planet from thousands of miles away, there are billions of stars around you, lighting up the darkness of innumerable galaxies in the most spectacular way.

Your stressor did not disappear, though from so far above the world that you know, it may feel like it for just a moment. The beauty and size of the universe around you can sometimes be enough to give you the perspective that you need. What may seem like an insurmountable challenge when you are sitting in it, is merely a small, fleeting blip when considered from the magnitude and glory of the galaxies surrounding us. Take a moment from this vantage point to take another deep, slow breath.

You may now begin to let go of this imaginary perspective, slowly, but gently floating back to earth, closer and closer to your body, until you are about to return. You are now close enough that you can see yourself again. Before you complete this journey, reflect on this feeling. No matter the stressor, it is but a small and fleeting moment that will come and go, barely noticed, among the hugeness of the cosmos. Now gently slip back into your body and take another deep, slow breath.

Everyone's stressors are different, and of course, when you are dealing with yours, it can be very difficult to say that it may not be such a big deal in the scheme of things. That is not really the purpose of this exercise. Everyone's stress is valid. The goal here is to allow you to see the issue from a bird's eye view, in the hopes of offering a better vantage point with which to assess your own situation. I hope that this tool is something that you can use often, and feel free to make it your own. Use your imagination to really delve deep into the perspective you need. Picture all of the colors and shapes and sensations of the environment around you to make it more real. Come back to this module as often as you like, or even take a few seconds during a particularly challenging time to view things from another angle.

Module 17: Happy Face

This module will bring us back to the concept of the neurochemical serotonin. Remember that we base some of our medical management of migraines on controlling the levels of this hormone in the body. Depression and anxiety are affected by this as well, and exacerbations of these problems are well-known triggers of headaches. The goal of this module is to promote mental imagery that can serve to increase the available serotonin in your mind. This will take advantage of the self-healing powers that your mind already possesses.

First, please find a quiet place and get into a comfortable position. Ideally, this will be a seated position with your feet flat and firmly placed on the ground, but pick any orientation that works for you. Relax your eyes and settle into the space around you. Feel how your body is in contact with the seat beneath you. Take a nice, deep breath. Relax the muscles of your face, your jaw, and the space between your eyes.

Search your mind for a happy memory, preferably recent, from the last few days to a week, but reaching into the more distant past is ok too. It could be something good that happened to you, praise from a respected colleague, or a pleasant experience with someone you really care about. Perhaps consider a really great and productive morning that you had to yourself. There is no wrong answer, just find something that truly made you happy and begin to focus on that moment. Probably the first memory that you thought of is the best one, but any will do.

Try to recall the way you felt when this was happening. What were you wearing at the time? Were you alone, or were you with someone? Was it hot outside, or was it cold? Was it raining, or perhaps it was sunny? Focusing on the details will help you bring yourself back to this moment and, if it feels right for you, allow your mouth to form a smile while you think of it. You may not feel like you're in the mood to smile right now, and that is ok. If you can manage even a small smile, that would be great, and if you can make it bigger, even better. Let it take over your face. Not just your lips, but bring your eyes into it as well. Feel how a little muscle movement on your face can start to have an effect in your mind.

Feel free to relax the muscles on your face, or keep smiling if it feels good, and enjoy the happy moment that you chose for just a few more seconds. Let its warmth envelop you and comfort you.

Ok, now again, let that smile creep back into the muscles of your face. Smaller at first, and then allow it to widen as much as you like. Keep holding on to the happy thought that you chose.

Again, allow the muscles of your face to relax. If you find that your thoughts have drifted, that's ok, just acknowledge that you are "thinking," and bring yourself back to your happy moment.

Now, for the final time, bring a smile back to your face. Let it grow as large as feels comfortable, and then allow it to relax.

Now, you may release your focus on this memory and bring yourself back to the present moment. Take a nice, deep breath. Though we may use pills to control serotonin, our body produces it naturally, and it fluctuates all the time based on our thoughts, experiences, and emotions. Going through the motions of expressing happiness with a physical smile, while guiding our minds with pleasant thoughts, can stimulate the production of serotonin. See if you can bring your mood to a better place, or improve your headache just a little, by finding a happy place in your mind and get a little boost of natural serotonin.

Module 18: Motivation

The goal of this module is to provide assistance with achieving your goals. We talked about all sorts of areas to improve our lives including exercise, diet, and sleep hygiene, but sometimes, it can seem really hard to get started on the right path. Finding the appropriate incentive to inspire you can be a challenge. I hope to guide you in discovering that encouragement within yourself.

Find a comfortable space, preferably in an upright, seated position, with your feet firmly planted in front of you. Keep your back and neck straight, and your chin up. Soften your eyes. Take a deep breath and relax. Ease the muscles around your face, your eyes, and unclench your jaw. For this module, you will focus on just one area in your life that needs a little bit of a push to get started, or to improve upon. Perhaps your goals include exercise or diet choices, or maybe it's simply being more confident. You can even focus on just being present more often. There is no right answer, and you can come back and do this again with any goal that you choose.

Relax your shoulders as well, but keep yourself in a position of confidence and alertness. Take another deep breath. Breathe in and out, paying attention to the way it makes your chest rise and fall.

Now, settle your focus on the goal for which you wish to motivate yourself. What is it about this goal that makes it so important to you? What will it help you to achieve? How will it improve your life? Will it *help you to feel better? Take a minute to pause here and really think about these questions.*

If you notice that your mind has wandered, just acknowledge, "thinking" and gently bring your attention back to your goals. Will this particular goal help you reach other objectives in your life as well? Will it benefit others, or just yourself? Understanding the reasons we do things can often be the intrinsic motivation we need to pursue our ambitions.

Picture yourself and your life after you have achieved this goal. What would it feel like to be in this position? Will you feel proud? Joy? Love? Put your feet in the shoes of this future self of yours and really try to experience what it may feel like to have achieved your goals.

Take a nice, deep breath. You may begin to release your focus on your goals and simply concentrate on your breathing for a moment longer.

Breathe in, and breathe out. Breathe in, and out. In, and out.

You can do anything that you put your mind to. Push yourself to your limits and you will find that suddenly the limits aren't what they once were. Every step forward opens more doors to you. Keep moving and one day you will look back and see that first line that you set for yourself way back in the distance. Be proud of yourself.

Module 19: Lovingkindness

Part of who we are inherently relies not only on how we perceive others, but on how others perceive us. This inextricable link is one of the main reasons why having a strong social support system is so important, both for addressing our pain, and for life. The goal of this module is to help build the feelings of interpersonal connection, which will provide you with a lifeline to the outside world. When you take the time to think of others in a warmhearted and generous manner, you will find that those feelings are returned to you in kind. It is essentially an investment in your own well-being. The better you feel on a day-to-day basis, the less stress and anxiety you will have. This can lead to less frequent and severe headaches, and will also place you in a better position to address your triggers.

Take a moment to find a comfortable space. Any position will do. Relax your eyes and take a nice, slow, deep breath. Soften the muscles around your eyes, your face, and your jaw. Straighten your neck and back.

Begin by paying attention to your breathing. Notice how your chest rises and falls with each breath.

Breathe in, your chest fills with air. Breathe out, and it settles back down. Breathe in, and breathe out. Breathe in, and out. In, and out.

Now, you can relax your attention on your breathing, and take a moment to choose someone to focus on for the first part of this lovingkindness exercise. The person should be someone whom you really care about. Someone who you may already love dearly. The first person you think of is probably ok. And if you want, come back and repeat this exercise with someone else in mind. There is no limit to the amount of love and kindness you can wish upon others.

Picture this person in your mind. Imagine that they are sitting or standing in front of you. It may be helpful to imagine what clothes they are wearing. What color is this person's hair, their eyes? Where were you when you last saw this person? Now, this next part may feel a little awkward if you have never tried this before, but at this point I would like you to silently speak this phrase while thinking about them.

"May this person be healthy. May this person be happy. May this person feel loved." Insert the name of the person you chose into the phrase.

"May _____ *be healthy. May* _____ *be happy. May* _____ *feel loved."*

Really focus your attention on the person that you chose. Bring them into your mind. Feel their warmth near you right now. Let the sensation of this love emanate from every cell of your being and out to them.

"May this person be healthy. May this person be happy. May this person feel loved."

Great. The second part of this module will be a little bit more challenging. At this point, you will choose another person to focus on. But this time, you will pick someone who you don't know very well. Perhaps someone at work, or the waiter at your favorite restaurant. Picture the details of his or her face. What were they wearing the last time you saw them? If you don't know this person's name, don't worry. Just use the phrase again.

"May this person be healthy. May this person be happy. May this person feel loved."

"May this person be healthy. May this person be happy. May this person feel loved."

"May this person be healthy. May this person be happy. May this person feel loved."

And now, you will shift your focus yet again. This time, you will attempt to take this sensation of lovingkindness, and focus it on yourself. This may be the most challenging part for many people and it may feel strange to think this way, but you deserve to feel loved and cared for.

"May I be healthy. May I be happy. May I feel loved."

"May I be healthy. May I be happy. May I feel loved."

"May I be healthy. May I be happy. May I feel loved."

Ok, you may begin to let go, and return your attention to your breathing again. Breathe in, and breathe out. Breathe in, and breathe out. Breathe in, and out.

How did it feel to focus goodness and love towards someone else? How did it feel when you focused that attention towards someone with whom you didn't have much prior experience? And finally, how did it feel when you turned that focus on yourself? Feel free to return to this exercise and try it out with a different focus of attention each time. I hope you take this experience with you, and remember to keep applying this love every day.

Module 20: Cooling Down

This short module is meant to create a healing atmosphere for your mind and body. We will again utilize the visualization powers of your imagination to provide some real pain relief. This module expands on the idea that my mother introduced me to years ago when I was a child in her arms suffering from my first migraine. There are so many other aspects to the healing process aside from medication alone. So, find a comfortable position – lying down is perfectly alright – in a nice quiet room if possible. Dim the lights if you can, and relax your eyes. Settle into this space and take a nice deep breath. As you breathe, pay attention to the way that your body is in contact with the surface beneath you. Let your breathing relax into its natural rhythm and notice the way it moves your chest and abdomen.

Envision a soft, wet cloth, saturated with icy, cold water. Imagine that dampness penetrating through the cloth, waiting to come into contact with your skin. Place it over your forehead, and begin to feel the cool, wet cloth caressing your face. Let the muscles of your forehead relax under its cold, gentle touch. Now focus on loosening the space between your eyes, your brow, and the area behind your eyes as well. Let them soften into a gently relaxed position.

Now imagine that the cloth is growing larger. It lightly brushes over your face and jaw. Let the coolness spread down and notice the muscles in those areas release as well. Unclench your jaw and open your mouth. Take another deep breath and feel the coolness of the air entering your mouth and nose. Follow it as it makes its way down to your lungs expanding your chest with its frosty flavor. Give yourself permission to let go of any pain or tension you might be feeling.

The coolness continues to spread. You notice the cold drifting down to your ears and neck, and feel the stress and muscles soften and calm there as well. It reaches all the way down to your shoulders now. Shrug them and feel the coldness spreading its healing powers up and down your body.

Take a moment to rest in this cool space for just a moment longer. Relax your attention on the cloth and coolness, and return to focus on your breathing. Gently breathing in and then breathing out. Take another deep breath and bring yourself back to this present moment. I hope that you feel somewhat relieved at this time. Please feel free to come back to this module anytime you need a little respite.

Closing Thoughts

Thank you so much for taking this journey with me. Mindfulness can be such a valuable resource for addressing pain and finding the right perspective. There is no wrong way to perform this skill. Just practice as regularly as you can, preferably every day, making it a part of your routine. Turning mindfulness into a habit, just like developing good sleep hygiene or a proper diet, can slowly but surely improve your symptoms. There are so many great products available for mindfulness, including apps, websites, journals, and books. Find a resource that you enjoy and you will be much more likely to stick with it. I would like to close by sharing five rules that I find to be most helpful in creating and maintaining positive change in my life.

1) *Maintain a positive outlook.*

This will not always be easy, but it will help you feel better, prevent migraines, and allow you to maintain the attitude you need to succeed. When you are feeling down, or suffering, remember to give yourself permission to see the light at the end of the tunnel. Commit yourself to changing your life for the better. Whether it's about committing to mindfulness, or to a healthier lifestyle involving dietary changes and physical exercise, push yourself to reach your goals. Once you achieve the initial set of objectives, make an effort to keep going and set new ones. This is why it is so important to maintain flexibility. My grandmother always used to say, "Man plans and God laughs." Even if you are not a religious person, one can easily see the relevance of this statement. We can set all the goals that we like, but somehow, something always seems to come up and interfere with our plans. Maintaining flexibility will allow you to find new ways to achieve your goals or to set new ones when the old goals are no longer relevant.

Even while you are struggling, it is so important to find the joy in each day. When I went back to college to complete the pre-med requirements for medical school, at first, I only thought about the ultimate objective of becoming an attending physician. But then, the idea of all of the steps in between, including medical school and residency began to get into my head. I quickly realized that focusing on the end goal was not going to be enough. I was getting frustrated and had periods of severe self-doubt. This was unsustainable, and I knew that I would fail if I did not change my perspective. You must learn to find the pleasure in every step of the process.

2) *Choose objectives that you will enjoy.*

When setting your goals, it is important that you can find joy in them. If it's exercise, choose a type that you actually want to do. If it's diet, pick something that you like, so that you can commit to a sustained change. If you pick something you really detest, you should not be surprised when you find yourself repeatedly avoiding it. This is true for exercise, diet choices, and mindfulness as well. The more pleasure you get out of it, the more likely it will play a role in your future success.

When I began to make exercise a more routine part of my life, I had a real problem motivating myself to do cardio. I really did not like running, and I found myself making excuses to avoid it all the time. So instead of just pushing on, I changed direction. I found that I enjoyed other cardio-based activities such as swimming and high-intensity interval training. That pleasure allowed me to pursue an activity that I knew would be good for my health, without being such an uphill battle. Be patient and give yourself adequate time and flexibility to make progress. Expect to encounter problems that you might not have considered. Challenges can arise from all areas, including from within. Some days, you may not feel like pushing forward. But put a smile on your face, straighten your back, stand tall, and you will achieve your goals.

3) *Take pride in your accomplishments.*

Whether you had one less cookie for dessert, or if you are celebrating 10 years of quitting smoking, it is important to give yourself credit. It is just as important to cut yourself some slack too. There will be many days where you don't feel like maintaining a strict diet, or you want a glass of wine with your dinner. And you may find that sometimes those decisions may lead directly or indirectly into triggering a headache. It's very easy to fall back on old habits like eating comfort foods, and making poor lifestyle choices. Don't give yourself a hard time for this. Life is hard enough. It is easy to feel discouraged in the face of any failure. But even the most successful people in the world stumble, often many times, before they succeed. I did not get an A in every class, nor did I know the answer to every question on every exam. I needed to push myself to my limits to get to where I am today. Be kind to yourself and take the opportunity to learn from your experiences.

4)   *Optimize your decision-making capabilities.*

While I pride myself on handling a lot of incoming information at a time in the emergency department, I am careful not to call it multi-tasking. We, as humans, are not really as skilled in this area as we would like to believe. Choose the focus of your attention at any given time, and hold it there until you are ready to move on. Just like in the emergency department, life calls upon us to make frequent decisions all the time. Some are important, like where to send your children to school, and how best to plan for retirement. Others are more mundane, such as what to eat for breakfast, or what shirt to wear. Each decision requires time, effort and valuable brain-power to perform.

Obviously, some of these decisions cannot be put off. However, some can be simplified. For example, you can create a menu of breakfast foods that you like and an order in which to eat them. This way, there is one less decision that you need to make every day. You can do the same for clothing, accessories, and many other areas of your life. This way, you won't get bogged down with the more mundane decisions and preserve the energy you need for the decisions that really count.

5) *Don't be afraid to ask for help.*

Whether from a family member, a supportive friend, or a professional, it is absolutely ok to ask for help. We are a social species. We depend on one another to assist us in times of need. Just by reaching out, you are already giving yourself a better chance of success. You are less likely to succumb to anxiety and depression, and more likely to stick with your goals if you have some accountability. Addressing chronic headache syndromes is likely a multi-modal approach. We have talked about lifestyle modifications such as diet, exercise, and sleep hygiene. Although we may not want to rely on them, pharmacological interventions are often needed for symptom relief and prevention. Perhaps most important of all is education, which can come in the form of consultations with headache specialists, reading, and discussions with friends or family going through the same thing. While keeping in mind that headaches and their triggers are complex, it is ok if some approaches work better for you. Find the interventions that work, and capitalize on them.

The social burden of headaches is difficult to calculate, but it is enormous. Taken cumulatively, there are likely millions of days of missed work and lost productivity worldwide due to headaches. There is a huge cost both to the healthcare system and to society as a result of diminished productivity. Even a small decrease in the number of headaches, if compounded, may result in drastic improvements. It is important to remember that you are not in this alone. There are so many of us that share the burden of this disease. Whether directly, like myself, or indirectly, like the public that suffers when we are unable to perform our jobs or require medical attention. Thus, the benefit of treatment and management is not solely for the individual, but for society as a whole. And remember, small steps can lead to dramatic and lasting changes in your life.

CITATIONS

1) Amin FM, Aristeidou S, Baraldi C, Czapinska-Ciepiela EK, Ariadni DD, Di Lenola D, Fenech C, Kampouris K, Karagiorgis G, Braschinsky M, Linde M; European Headache Federation School of Advanced Studies (EHF-SAS). "The association between migraine and physical exercise." J Headache Pain. 2018 Sep 10;19(1):83. doi: 10.1186/s10194-018-0902-y. PMID: 30203180; PMCID: PMC6134860.

2) Arca, K.N., Halker Singh, R.B. *The Hypertensive Headache: a Review.* Curr Pain Headache Rep 23, 30 (2019). https://doi.org/10.1007/s11916-019-0767-z

3) Albanês Oliveira Bernardo A, Lys Medeiros F, Sampaio Rocha-Filho PA. "Osmophobia and Odor-Triggered Headaches in Children and Adolescents: Prevalence, Associated Factors, and Importance in the Diagnosis of Migraine." Headache. 2020 May;60(5):954-966. doi: 10.1111/head.13806. Epub 2020 Apr 15. PMID: 32293736.

4) Barber M, Pace A. "Exercise and Migraine Prevention: a Review of the Literature." Curr Pain Headache Rep. 2020 Jun 11;24(8):39. doi: 10.1007/s11916-020-00868-6. PMID: 32529311.

5) Bektas, H., Karabulut, H., Doganay, B. et al. "Allergens might trigger migraine attacks." Acta Neurol Belg 117, 91–95 (2017). https://doi-org.ezproxy.med.nyu.edu/10.1007/s13760-016-0645-y

6) Beuthin J, Veronesi M, Grosberg B, Evans RW. "Gluten-Free Diet and Migraine." Headache. 2020 Nov;60(10):2526-2529. doi: 10.1111/head.13993. Epub 2020 Oct 6. PMID: 33022759.

7) Bird SR, Hawley JA. "Update on the effects of physical activity on insulin sensitivity in humans." BMJ Open Sport & Exercise Medicine 2017;2:e000143. doi: 10.1136/bmjsem-2016-000143

8) Burch RC, Buse DC, Lipton RB. "Migraine: Epidemiology, Burden, and Comorbidity." Neurol Clin. 2019 Nov;37(4):631-649. doi: 10.1016/j.ncl.2019.06.001. Epub 2019 Aug 27. PMID: 31563224.

9) Calhoun AH. "Understanding Menstrual Migraine." Headache. 2018 Apr;58(4):626-630. doi: 10.1111/head.13291. Epub 2018 Mar 1. PMID: 29492961.

10) Carvalho GF, Schwarz A, Szikszay TM, Adamczyk WM, Bevilaqua-Grossi D, Luedtke K. "Physical therapy and migraine: musculoskeletal and balance dysfunctions and their relevance for clinical practice." Braz J Phys Ther. 2020 Jul-Aug;24(4):306-317. doi: 10.1016/j.bjpt.2019.11.001. Epub 2019 Nov 29. PMID: 31813696; PMCID: PMC7351966.

11) Choi CY. "Chronic pain and opiate management." Dis Mon. 2016 Sep;62(9):334-45. doi: 10.1016/j.disamonth.2016.05.013. PMID: 27569588.

12) Chunhua X, Jiacui D, Xue L, Kai W. "Impaired emotional memory and decision-making following primary insomnia. » Medicine (Baltimore). 2019 Jul;98(29):e16512. doi: 10.1097/MD.0000000000016512. PMID: 31335727; PMCID: PMC6709269.

13) Clark I, Landolt HP. "Coffee, caffeine, and sleep: A systematic review of epidemiological studies and randomized controlled trials." Sleep Med Rev. 2017 Feb;31:70-78. doi: 10.1016/j.smrv.2016.01.006. Epub 2016 Jan 30. PMID: 26899133.

14) Cortelli P, Grimaldi D, Guaraldi P, Pierangeli G. "Headache and hypertension." Neurol Sci. 2004 Oct;25 Suppl 3:S132-4. doi: 10.1007/s10072-004-0271-y. PMID: 15549522.

15) Delpont B, Blanc C, Osseby GV, Hervieu-Bègue M, Giroud M, Béjot Y. "Pain after stroke: A review." Rev Neurol (Paris). 2018 Dec;174(10):671-674. doi: 10.1016/j.neurol.2017.11.011. Epub 2018 Jul 24. PMID: 30054011.

16) Ebrahim, I.O., Shapiro, C.M., Williams, A.J. and Fenwick, P.B. (2013), "Alcohol and Sleep I: Effects on Normal Sleep." Alcohol Clin Exp Res, 37: 539`-549. https://doi.org/10.1111/acer.12006

17) Edvinsson L. (2019) "Role of CGRP in Migraine." In: Brain S., Geppetti P. (eds) Calcitonin Gene-Related Peptide (CGRP) Mechanisms. Handbook of Experimental Pharmacology, vol 255. Springer, Cham. https://doi.org/10.1007/164_2018_201

18) Friedman BW, Mistry B, West JR, Wollowitz A. "The association between headache and elevated blood pressure among patients presenting to an ED." Am J Emerg Med. 2014 Sep;32(9):976-81. doi: 10.1016/j.ajem.2014.05.017. Epub 2014 May 20. PMID: 24993684.

19) Gaul C, Liesering-Latta E, Schäfer B, Fritsche G, Holle D. "Integrated multidisciplinary care of headache disorders: A narrative review." Cephalalgia. 2016 Oct;36(12):1181-1191. doi: 10.1177/0333102415617413. Epub 2016 Jul 11. PMID: 26646785.

20) Gu Q, Hou JC, Fang XM. "Mindfulness Meditation for Primary Headache Pain: A Meta-Analysis." Chin Med J (Engl). 2018;131(7):829-838. doi:10.4103/0366-6999.228242

21) Haghighi FS, Rahmanian M, Namiranian N, Arzaghi SM, Dehghan F, Chavoshzade F, Sepehri F. "Migraine and type 2 diabetes; is there any association?" J Diabetes Metab Disord. 2016 Sep 8;15(1):37. doi: 10.1186/s40200-016-0241-y. PMID: 27617234; PMCID: PMC5016935.

22) Hansen AP, Marcussen NS, Klit H, Andersen G, Finnerup NB, Jensen TS. "Pain following stroke: a prospective study." Eur J Pain. 2012 Sep;16(8):1128-36. doi: 10.1002/j.1532-2149.2012.00123.x. Epub 2012 Mar 9. PMID: 22407963.

23) Goadsby PJ. "Pathophysiology of migraine." Ann Indian Acad Neurol. 2012;15(Suppl 1):S15-S22. doi:10.4103/0972-2327.99993

24) Guo XN, Lu JJ, Ni JQ, Lu HF, Zhao HR, Chen G. "The role of oxygen in cluster headache." Med Gas Res. 2019 Oct-Dec;9(4):229-231. doi: 10.4103/2045-9912.273961. PMID: 31898608; PMCID: PMC7802413.

25) Irby MB, Bond DS, Lipton RB, Nicklas B, Houle TT, Penzien DB. "Aerobic Exercise for Reducing Migraine Burden: Mechanisms, Markers, and Models of Change Processes." Headache. 2016 Feb;56(2):357-69. doi: 10.1111/head.12738. Epub 2015 Dec 8. PMID: 26643584; PMCID: PMC4813301.

26) Islam MA, Amin MN, Siddiqui SA, Hossain MP, Sultana F, Kabir MR. "Trans fatty acids and lipid profile: A serious risk factor to cardio-vascular disease, cancer and diabetes." Diabetes Metab Syndr. 2019 Mar-Apr;13(2):1643-1647. doi: 10.1016/j.dsx.2019.03.033. Epub 2019 Mar 16. PMID: 31336535.

27) Juliano LM, Kardel PG, Harrell PT, Muench C, Edwards KC. "Investigating the role of expectancy in caffeine withdrawal using the balanced placebo design." Hum Psychopharmacol. 2019 Mar;34(2):e2692. doi: 10.1002/hup.2692. Epub 2019 Mar 12. PMID: 30861208.

28) Khazaei, M., Hosseini Nejad Mir, N., Yadranji Aghdam, F. et al. "Effectiveness of intravenous dexamethasone, metoclopramide, ketoro-lac, and chlorpromazine for pain relief and prevention of recurrence in the migraine headache: a prospective double-blind randomized clini-cal trial." Neurol Sci 40, 1029–1033 (2019). https://doi.org/10.1007/s10072-019-03766-x

29) Klinzing JG, Niethard N, Born J. "Mechanisms of systems memory consolidation during sleep." Nat Neurosci. 2019 Oct;22(10):1598-1610. doi: 10.1038/s41593-019-0467-3. Epub 2019 Aug 26. Erratum in: Nat Neurosci. 2019 Sep 11;: PMID: 31451802.

30) Knab, A, Shanely, R., Corbin, K., Jin, F., Sha, W., Nieman, D. A. "45-Minute Vigorous Exercise Bout Increases Metabolic Rate for 14 Hours." Med Sci Sports Exerc. 2011;43(9):1643-1648. doi:10.1249/ MSS.0b013e3182118891.

31) Kojić Z, Stojanović D. "Pathophysiology of migraine--from molecular to personalized medicine." Med Pregl. 2013 Jan-Feb;66(1-2):53-7. doi: 10.2298/mpns1302053k. PMID: 23534301.

32) Lemmens J, De Pauw J, Van Soom T, Michiels S, Versijpt J, van Breda E, Castien R, De Hertogh W. "The effect of aerobic exercise on the number of migraine days, duration and pain intensity in migraine: a systematic literature review and meta-analysis." J Headache Pain. 2019 Feb 14;20(1):16. doi: 10.1186/s10194-019-0961-8. PMID: 30764753; PMCID: PMC6734345.

33) Li G, Li J, Gao F. "Exercise and Cardiovascular Protection." Adv Exp Med Biol. 2020;1228:205-216. doi: 10.1007/978-981-15-1792-1_14. PMID: 32342460.

34) Li W, Bertisch SM, Mostofsky E, Buettner C, Mittleman MA. "Weather, ambient air pollution, and risk of migraine headache onset among patients with migraine." Environ Int. 2019 Nov;132:105100. doi: 10.1016/j. envint.2019.105100. Epub 2019 Aug 22. PMID: 31446321; PMCID: PMC7523027.

35) Ljubisavljevic S, Zidverc Trajkovic J. "Cluster headache: pathophysiology, diagnosis and treatment." J Neurol. 2019 May;266(5):1059-1066. doi: 10.1007/s00415-018-9007-4. Epub 2018 Aug 17. PMID: 30120560.

36) Maini K, Schuster NM. "Headache and Barometric Pressure: a Narrative Review." Curr Pain Headache Rep. 2019 Nov 9;23(11):87. doi: 10.1007/ s11916-019-0826-5. PMID: 31707623.

37) Martin VT, Vij B. "Diet and Headache: Part 1." Headache. 2016 Oct;56(9):1543-1552. doi: 10.1111/head.12953. PMID: 27699780.

38) Nestoriuc Y, Martin A, Rief W, Andrasik F. "Biofeedback treatment for headache disorders: a comprehensive efficacy review." Appl Psychophysiol

Biofeedback. 2008 Sep;33(3):125-40. doi: 10.1007/s10484-008-9060-3. Epub 2008 Aug 26. PMID: 18726688.

39) Nery C, Moraes SRA, Novaes KA, Bezerra MA, Silveira PVC, Lemos A. "Effectiveness of resistance exercise compared to aerobic exercise without insulin therapy in patients with type 2 diabetes mellitus: a meta-analysis." Braz J Phys Ther. 2017 Nov-Dec;21(6):400-415. doi: 10.1016/j.bjpt.2017.06.004. Epub 2017 Jul 5. PMID: 28728958; PMCID: PMC5693273.

40) Obayashi Y, Nagamura Y. "Does monosodium glutamate really cause headache? : a systematic review of human studies." J Headache Pain. 2016;17:54. doi:10.1186/s10194-016-0639-4

41) Olesen J. "The role of nitric oxide (NO) in migraine, tension-type headache and cluster headache." Pharmacol Ther. 2008 Nov;120(2):157-71. doi: 10.1016/j.pharmthera.2008.08.003. Epub 2008 Aug 23. PMID: 18789357.

42) Ong, J.J.Y., Wei, D.YT. & Goadsby, P.J. "Recent Advances in Pharmacotherapy for Migraine Prevention: From Pathophysiology to New Drugs." Drugs 78, 411–437 (2018). https://doi.org/10.1007/s40265-018-0865-y

43) Pattison, K. "Worker, interrupted: the cost of task switching." Fast Company. 28 Jul 2008. Web. Accessed March 17, 2021. https://www.fastcompany.com/944128/worker-interrupted-cost-task-switching

44) Peixoto AJ. "Acute Severe Hypertension." N Engl J Med. 2019 Nov 7;381(19):1843-1852. doi: 10.1056/NEJMcp1901117. PMID: 31693807.

45) Peres MFP, Mercante JPP, Tobo PR, Kamei H, Bigal ME. "Anxiety and depression symptoms and migraine: a symptom-based approach research." J Headache Pain. 2017 Dec;18(1):37. doi: 10.1186/s10194-017-0742-1. Epub 2017 Mar 21. PMID: 28324317; PMCID: PMC5360747.

46) Pérez-Muñoz A, Buse DC, Andrasik F. "Behavioral Interventions for Migraine." Neurol Clin. 2019 Nov;37(4):789-813. doi: 10.1016/j.ncl.2019.07.003. Epub 2019 Aug 22. PMID: 31563233.

47) Probyn K, Bowers H, Mistry D, Caldwell F, Underwood M, Patel S, Sandhu HK, Matharu M, Pincus T; CHESS team. "Non-pharmacological self-management for people living with migraine or tension-type headache: a systematic review including analysis of intervention components." BMJ Open. 2017 Aug 11;7(8):e016670. doi: 10.1136/bmjopen-2017-016670. PMID: 28801425; PMCID: PMC5629643.

48) Robbins MS, Robertson CE, Kaplan E, Ailani J, Charleston L 4th, Kuruvilla D, Blumenfeld A, Berliner R, Rosen NL, Duarte R, Vidwan J, Halker RB, Gill N, Ashkenazi A. "The Sphenopalatine Ganglion: Anatomy, Pathophysiology, and Therapeutic Targeting in Headache." Headache. 2016 Feb;56(2):240-58. doi: 10.1111/head.12729. Epub 2015 Nov 30. PMID: 26615983.

49) Sacks FM, Lichtenstein AH, Wu JHY, Appel LJ, Creager MA, Kris-Etherton PM, Miller M, Rimm EB, Rudel LL, Robinson JG, Stone NJ, Van Horn LV; American Heart Association. "Dietary Fats and Cardiovascular Disease: A Presidential Advisory From the American Heart Association." Circulation. 2017 Jul 18;136(3):e1-e23. doi: 10.1161/CIR.0000000000000510. Epub 2017 Jun 15. Erratum in: Circulation. 2017 Sep 5;136(10):e195. PMID: 28620111.

50) Schulte, L.H., Jürgens, T.P. & May, A. "Photo-, osmo- and phono-phobia in the premonitory phase of migraine: mistaking symptoms for triggers?" J Headache Pain 16, 14 (2015). https://doi.org/10.1186/s10194-015-0495-7

51) Seminowicz DA, Burrowes SAB, Kearson A, Zhang J, Krimmel SR, Samawi L, Furman AJ, Keaser ML, Gould NF, Magyari T, White L, Goloubeva O, Goyal M, Peterlin BL, Haythornthwaite JA. "Enhanced mindfulness-based stress reduction in episodic migraine: a randomized clinical trial with magnetic resonance imaging outcomes." Pain. 2020 Aug;161(8):1837-1846. doi: 10.1097/j.pain.0000000000001860. Epub 2020 Mar 13. PMID: 32701843; PMCID: PMC7487005.

52) Shafqat R, Flores-Montanez Y, Delbono V, Nahas SJ. "Updated Evaluation of IV Dihydroergotamine (DHE) for Refractory Migraine:

Patient Selection and Special Considerations." J Pain Res. 2020;13:859-864. Published 2020 Apr 30. doi:10.2147/JPR.S203650

53) Silva, Miguel, et al. "Sulfite concentration and the occurrence of headache in young adults: a prospective study." European Journal of Clinical Nutrition, vol. 73, no. 9, 2019, p. 1316. Gale OneFile: Health and Medicine, link.gale.com/apps/doc/A598451181/HRCA?u=nysl_me_nyuniv&sid=HRCA&xid=d588436c. Accessed 10 Mar. 2021.

54) Skaugset LM, Farrell S, Carney M, Wolff M, Santen SA, Perry M, Cico SJ. "Can You Multitask? Evidence and Limitations of Task Switching and Multitasking in Emergency Medicine." Ann Emerg Med. 2016 Aug;68(2):189-95. doi: 10.1016/j.annemergmed.2015.10.003. Epub 2015 Nov 14. PMID: 26585046.

55) Song TJ, Cho SJ, Kim WJ, Yang KI, Yun CH, Chu MK. "Poor sleep quality in migraine and probable migraine: a population study." J Headache Pain. 2018 Jul 25;19(1):58. doi: 10.1186/s10194-018-0887-6. PMID: 30046921; PMCID: PMC6060206.

56) Sutherland HG, Albury CL, Griffiths LR. "Advances in genetics of migraine." J Headache Pain. 2019 Jun 21;20(1):72. doi: 10.1186/s10194-019-1017-9. PMID: 31226929; PMCID: PMC6734342.

57) Tang J, Gibson SJ. "A psychophysical evaluation of the relationship between trait anxiety, pain perception, and induced state anxiety." J Pain. 2005 Sep;6(9):612-9. doi: 10.1016/j.jpain.2005.03.009. PMID: 16139780.

58) Van Dam NT, van Vugt MK, Vago DR, et al. "Mind the Hype: A Critical Evaluation and Prescriptive Agenda for Research on Mindfulness and Meditation," [published correction appears in Perspect Psychol Sci. 2020 Sep;15(5):1289-1290]. Perspect Psychol Sci. 2018;13(1):36-61. doi:10.1177/1745691617709589

59) Vetvik KG, MacGregor EA. "Sex differences in the epidemiology, clinical features, and pathophysiology of migraine." Lancet Neurol. 2017

Jan;16(1):76-87. doi: 10.1016/S1474-4422(16)30293-9. Epub 2016 Nov 9. PMID: 27836433.

60) Vitale KC, Owens R, Hopkins SR, Malhotra A. "Sleep Hygiene for Optimizing Recovery in Athletes: Review and Recommendations." Int J Sports Med. 2019 Aug;40(8):535-543. doi: 10.1055/a-0905-3103. Epub 2019 Jul 9. PMID: 31288293; PMCID: PMC6988893.

61) Wakerley BR. "Medication-overuse headache." Pract Neurol. 2019 Oct;19(5):399-403. doi: 10.1136/practneurol-2018-002048. Epub 2019 Jul 4. PMID: 31273078.

62) Wells RE, O'Connell N, Pierce CR, et al. « Effectiveness of Mindfulness Meditation vs Headache Education for Adults With Migraine: A Randomized Clinical Trial." JAMA Intern Med. Published online December 14, 2020. doi:10.1001/jamainternmed.2020.7090

63) Wood B, Rea MS, Plitnick B, Figueiro MG. "Light level and duration of exposure determine the impact of self-luminous tablets on melatonin suppression." Appl Ergon. 2013 Mar;44(2):237-40. doi: 10.1016/j.apergo.2012.07.008. Epub 2012 Jul 31. PMID: 22850476.

64) Yerkes, R. M., & Dodson, J. D. (1908). "The relation of strength of stimulus to rapidity of habit-formation." Journal of Comparative Neurology and Psychology, 18(5), 459–482.